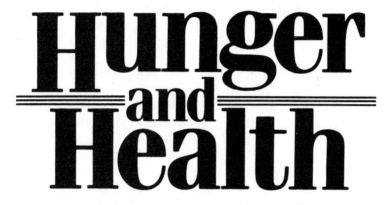

Hunger and Health

Eleven Key Questions on Farming, Food, and Health in the Third World

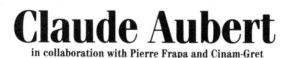

Claude Aubert

in collaboration with Pierre Frapa and Cinam-Gret

Translated by Camille J. Cusumano, Wendy Greenberg, and Nicholas Bellotto

Rodale Press, Emmaus, Pennsylvania

Original title: *Onze Questions Cles sur l'Agriculture, l'Alimentation, la Sante, le Tiers-monde*, © Terre Vivante, Paris, 1983. ISBN 2-904082-02-6

English translation © 1985, Rodale Press, Inc.

The translators wish to thank Heather Danton for her invaluable contribution to the editing of the translated text.

Book design: Linda Jacopetti
Chart preparation: Darla L. Hoffman

Library of Congress Cataloging in Publication Data
Aubert, Claude, 1944-
    Hunger and health.

    Translation of: Onze questions clés sur l'agriculture, l'alimentation, la santé, le Tiers-monde.
    Bibliography: p.
    Includes index.
    1. Agriculture—developing countries—Addresses, essays, lectures. 2. Food supply—Developing countries—Addresses, essays, lectures. 3. Public health—Developing countries—Addresses, essays, lectures. 4. Malnutrition—Developing countries—Prevention—Addresses, essays, lectures. 5. Food crops—Developing countries—Addresses, essays, lectures. 6. Agricultural chemicals—Developing countries—Addresses, essays, lectures. 7. Diet—Developing countries—Addresses, essays, lectures. 8. Food industry and trade—Developing countries—Addresses, essays, lectures. I. Frapa, Pierre. II. CINAM-GRET (Working group) III. Title. IV. Title: Eleven key questions on farming, food, and health in the Third World [DNLM: 1. Agriculture—methods. 2. Developing Countries. 3. Environmental Health. 4. Food Supply. 5. Nutrition Disorders—prevention & control. WA 695 A889o]
S482.A9313   1985   363.8′09172′4   85-10733
ISBN 0-87857-549-9 hardcover

2   4   6   8   10   9   7   5   3   1   hardcover

Contents

Foreword

This work obviously does not claim to have miraculous solutions to farming, food, and health problems in the Third World. Its goals are more modest: to ask questions, to show the inadequacy of typical answers, and to offer simple, creative, low-cost alternatives that avoid pollution and pose no health risks.

But we must be wary of thinking that there is a simple, cheap technology that is "appropriate" for Third World countries and a higher technology for industrialized countries. The solutions we propose are of concern to rich countries as well. It is significant that they have been adopted by a small but growing segment of the population in Europe and the United States.

There are, in fact, two kinds of technologies: those that aid mankind and those that do not. The destruction of humus, the decline in food quality, and the rise in health hazards, pollution, and unemployment are universal ills, often brought on by technologies developed in Western countries.

It will sooner or later be necessary for all countries to begin adopting the principles set forth in this book. This choice may not seem so urgent and necessary in the industrialized countries as in others, but let's not fool ourselves: "appropriate technologies" will develop in the Third World only to the degree rich countries gradually adopt them.

It's not only a question of technology: it is also necessary to change our eating habits and our way of living. It is only if we agree—before we are forced to do so by future events—to consume fewer unnecessary goods, to reestablish a balance between city and country, and to restore a place to farming and small-scale industry that we will really help the Third World countries resolve their problems and, at the same time, our own. This will take time, for it will be necessary to win over the people and their leaders before a new type of society can be built. The sooner we put ourselves to this task, the greater will be our chances of wiping out malnutrition in the Third World—as well as our chances of saving our own society, which is sicker and more threatened than it appears.

Introduction

In many developing countries, food problems are serious and getting worse all the time. Crop yields are very low, storage losses are high, and export crops take precedence over food crops. The state of health of the lowest social classes in certain countries is appalling.

Food assistance, useful as a stopgap measure, brings no permanent solution—it does just the opposite, in fact. It aggravates inequities, discourages the small farmer, and reaches only a fraction of those who really need food assistance as it forces them into a state of dependence. In the hands of rich countries, finally, food assistance becomes a political weapon.

Clearly, each country's goal is to be capable of nourishing its population with its own resources, that is, to supply enough food containing the necessary nutrients. The usual ways of achieving this goal rely upon the technologies used in industrialized countries, where sophisticated farming and food production techniques—those that seemed so remarkably effective at first—were developed.

Simultaneously, the higher life expectancy in these countries might lead to the conclusion that their diets are nutritionally satisfying.

Today, in spite of these results, it is clear that the agricultural production systems and eating habits of industrialized countries will be harmful in the long run. There are several reasons for this.

1. *They can never be applied to the entire world.*
   They constitute an enormous waste of energy, land, and natural resources. The industrialized countries can afford them for now, but these countries are depleting other countries' riches for their own benefit. From an energy point of view alone, the American food system would exhaust the world's entire petroleum reserves in several decades.
2. *They often have disastrous consequences on soil fertility and the environment.*
   The farming techniques of industrialized countries frequently lead to impoverishment of the soil's humus and almost always the pollution of soil, water, food—even the entire ecosystem—with pesticides or nitrates.
3. *They are harmful to human health.*
   In Western countries, poor eating habits are becoming a major cause of the increased death rate from cancer and heart disease. Eventually, the Western diet may lead to decreased life expectancy.

The purposes of this book are:

1. To draw attention to problems caused by modern techniques of food production and processing and by our diet.
2. To make known the results obtained through food production methods that promote autonomy—methods that are less polluting, that respect the ecosystem, and that yield food conforming to human needs.
3. To point out the areas where research work is needed so that the producers' needs, the balance of the ecosystem over time, and the production of healthy food are all assured.

In the following pages we will mainly discuss the technical aspects of the questions raised. This does not mean that we are dismissing the cultural, sociological, and political aspects: they must obviously be taken into account before any solution is implemented.

Question 1

Can agricultural production in the Third World be increased without increasing the use of chemical fertilizers and pesticides?

Agricultural production must be increased to solve the problem of malnutrition, but what will be the cost to our economy and environment? Among the available means for increasing agricultural production, chemical fertilizers and pesticides figure prominently in development programs. But we must often pay dearly for the increased production that they permit. The majority of developing countries must import fertilizers, often to the detriment of their balance of trade. The construction of fertilizer factories makes a reduction in imports possible but requires large investments. Because of their cost, fertilizers are often reserved for export crops so domestically consumed crops rarely benefit from them. Moreover, the poorest farmers cannot afford to buy fertilizer, or they do so at great cost, making them even poorer.

Long-term misuse of fertilizers leads to depletion of the soil's humus, mineral imbalances, and sometimes an actual lowering of crop yields. Fertilizers, notably nitrates, in high quantities contribute to water pollution and have negative effects on food quality (see Question 3). Mineral fertilizers are often poorly balanced and provide no means of organic restoration. Therefore, in spite of their spectacular short-term effects, mineral fertilizers bring no worthwhile solution (Fleury and Mollard, 1976). This conclusion is highlighted by the fact that fertilizer production also consumes high amounts of energy, requiring approximately two barrels of oil per barrel of nitrogen fertilizer (Fevrier and Poly, 1979).

1

Pesticides present serious dangers for users while they pollute food, water, and the environment (see Question 3) (Dajoz, 1969; ACTA and CoLuMa, 1977). Knowledgeable pesticide use presupposes a level of technology that many farmers in developing countries will not be able to acquire quickly. Cost-effectiveness of pesticide use is also a question, since use of pesticides may require multiple treatments. Because of the pesticides, plants become vulnerable to new parasites, as these parasites' natural enemies are destroyed by the treatments. The pests themselves become resistant to pesticides so that farmers must continually seek new products to control them (FAO, 1977; Delwaulle, 1973). It is common to see cotton plantations receive 15 to 20 insecticide treatments. Some vegetable crops, and especially fruit crops (grapes, apples), receive 20, 30, and sometimes 35 treatments in a single season.

It is possible to obtain higher agricultural yields while limiting the use of chemical fertilizers and pesticides. A lasting increase in yields occurs through improved soil fertility, that is, through an increase in the soil's humus content and biological activity, accompanied by correction of mineral deficiencies (Egger, 1980). Simple techniques requiring no purchase from outside sources, such as recycling of organic matter, composting, crop association, crop rotations, natural fertilizers, and mulching, aid in improving soil fertility (Aubert, 1977; Sedogoetal, 1979; Egger, 1980; Collombon, 1980). Mineral deficiencies can often be corrected simply by crushing local products such as natural phosphates, dolomites, and limestone. When animal wastes, farming and food industry residues, and household garbage are recycled, large quantities of organic matter, important to the soil as a source of fertilizing elements and humus, are restored.

Many parasites can be combated without recourse to chemical pesticides. Recent research has demonstrated that frequency and gravity of parasite attacks depend directly on the physiological state of cultivated plants (Chaboussou, 1974 and 1980). As a rule, a strong correlation exists between the seriousness of parasite attacks and the amount of soluble substances (nonprotein nitrogen and sugar) present in the plants. The accumulation of soluble substances results from a physiological imbalance, specifically, a slowing down of protein synthesis. This is aggravated by numerous pesticides (insecticides, fungicides, herbicides), by fertilization imbalances (excessive nitrogen, mineral deficiencies), by working the soil under poor conditions, or by choosing plant varieties that are not adapted to the climate.

Numerous observations made by practitioners of organic farming methods have confirmed that plants cultivated in balanced soil with good biological activity are much less frequently attacked by parasites than the same plants cultivated in imbalanced soil that is poor in humus (Aubert, 1977). Nontoxic means for fighting parasites also exist. Certain crop associations result in a significant reduction in parasite attacks. Biological pest control has already given us some very interesting applications, such as the use of *Bacillus thuringiensis* against caterpillars, or trichogramma wasps against the meal-moth. In both Russia and China, biological pest control techniques are used on a large scale (Taylor, 1977; Augst, 1981; Franz, 1983; OCDE, 1977). Plant-based insecticides (pyrethrum, rotenone, quassia) have a low toxicity, yet they are very effective and can be manufactured locally in many parts of the developing world. It is therefore possible, contrary to widespread opinion, to cut down the use of pesticides considerably without harming production.

It is interesting to note that agricultural methods that avoid the use of chemical fertilizers, pesticides, and limited energy sources are exciting more and more interest in industrialized countries. These low-input methodologies are being practiced by an increasing number of farmers both in developed and developing countries. In June 1980, the United States Department of Agriculture (USDA) published a report that was highly in favor of organic farming. The authors of the report concluded that this type of agriculture brings positive solutions to the problems posed by conventional agriculture (pollution, soil erosion, excessive consumption of energy) and that there should be help for farmers who want to practice organic farming (USDA, 1980). There are also research programs on organic farming in several European countries (France, Switzerland, the Netherlands, Germany).

Supplementary Readings for Question 1

Can agricultural production in the Third World be increased without increasing the use of chemical fertilizers and pesticides?

Economic Limitations for Fertilizer Use

From 1951 to 1966, nitrate fertilizer consumption increased 146 percent throughout the world, while agricultural yields increased only 34 percent. Nitrogen-fixing bacteria are killed when high levels of nitrates are introduced into the soil, increasing the amount of nitrates necessary to raise or just to maintain production levels. Already in the United States' grain belt, the land's production ceiling is being reached. To maintain productivity each year, it is necessary to continue or increase the use of nitrates. Today 1.2 billion tons of grain are produced worldwide annually. (To feed all humanity on a survival level, 800 million would suffice. For all humanity to have a Western-style diet, it would be necessary to produce almost double that by the year 2000.) At present, 80 million tons of artificial fertilizers are consumed each year, yet this satisfies only one-fifth of the demand for nitrogen fertilizer. It would take about 200 factories capable of producing a half million barrels of fertilizer a year to fulfill the demand for artificial nitrates.

Excerpted from: *Conti, L. "Qu'est ce que l'écologie?" ("What Is Ecology?") Petite Collection Maspéro, no. 300, Paris, 1978, p. 157. Original title: "Che cos'è l'ecologia," Gabriele Mazzotta, Milan.*

A Fertilizer Factory in Every Village

Consider, for example, the case of fertilizer, which can be produced synthetically from oil or coal, or organically as stabilized sludge from the anaerobic microbial fermentation of sewage and cattle wastes. Ruling out oil-based fertilizer plants, in view of the total inadequacy of crude from indigenous production in petroleum-importing developing countries and the rapidly escalating price of imported crude, one can compare the production of 230,000 tons per year of nitrogen in large-scale coal-based fertilizer plants of the type being planned in India, and in village-scale biogas fertilizer plants.

Table 1-1   Production of 230,000 tons of nitrogen per year by Western and alternative technologies

	Western technology	Alternative technology
Number of plants	1	26,150 (at 8.8 tons per year per plant)
Capital cost	about $140 million	about $125 million (at $4,825 per plant)
Foreign exchange	about $70 million	nil
Capital/sales ratio (at $510 per ton nitrogen)	1.20	1.07
Employment	1,000	130,750 (at 5 per plant)
Energy	about 0.1 million MWh per year *consumption*	6.35 million MWh per year *generation*

It is obvious from table 1–1 that the adoption of the alternative biofertilizer technology will result in the dispersal of production to 26,150 villages, rather than concentrate it in one center; save $15 million of precious capital in a capital-poor country; conserve $70 million of foreign exchange in the midst of balance-of-payments problems; yield a much higher rate of return on investment; generate 130 times more employment; provide employment to the rural poor rather than the urban elite; produce fertilizer where it is consumed, and therefore relieve the burden on the struggling transport system; reduce unnecessary overheads on packaging, transport, marketing, and advertising; and protect villagers from the private and government apparatus set up to take fertilizer from the urban factory to the village consumers.

In addition, the smaller plants usually have much shorter gestation times and can be brought to full capacity in a matter of months compared to the years required for large plants.

The type of village-scale biogas fertilizer plants envisaged can play a crucial role in promoting village self-reliance with respect to fertilizer requirements. For instance, in the case of India, the biofertilizer output of each village-scale plant can service the average cropped-land area of 290 hectares per village with about two-and-a-half times the present level of nitrogen consumption, which is about 12 kilograms per hectare. And this dramatic increase can be achieved by anaerobically fermenting the village wastes from 500 human beings and 250 cattle (assuming 75 percent collection efficiency), i.e., by relying on locally available renewable resources.

Excerpted from: *Reddy, A. K. N. "Le cheval de Troie" ("The Trojan Horse") Cérès, no. 50, March-April 1976, pp. 42-43.*

Fertilization and Soil Conservation

The abuse of chemical fertilizers pollutes water, alters plant composition and, over time, depletes the soil of humus. Moreover, intensive fertilizer use permanently decreases the soil's nutritive potential. Even if the plants absorb large amounts of nutritive elements, the farmer, who desires maximum production and finds available cheap fertilizers, expects the excess to leach. If this does not happen, the accumulated fertilizers can drastically alter plant composition, resulting in a concentration of noxious substances within the plants (Agarwal, 1978). If leaching occurs, the water becomes contaminated with these substances.

Not only are these fertilizers hazardous to health, but we must even question their ability to fertilize in light of the physical changes that may ensue in soil structure. Certain authors have reported a rapid decline of organic matter in the soil and a degeneration of its physical structure in experimental samples treated solely with chemical fertilizers. They conclude that a new set of circumstances has developed in which nitrates are not delivered to the plant in an optimal way. Part of the nitrogen brought to the soil is either broken down or lost through leaching (Fleury and Mollard, 1976). B. Commoner demonstrates that when an excessive amount of nitrates is introduced in grain-growing regions, a large amount is not retained by the plants. In the United States, 50 to 80 percent of nitrate fertilizers are actually absorbed by crops. In terms of energy alone, this represents a great waste.

One of the chief concerns about use of chemical fertilizers is the loss of humus in intensively cultivated regions. This problem first appeared in colonial territories, notably in Algeria, where 80 percent of the humus was destroyed after 100 years of colonial agriculture, and it occurs today in all heavily agricultural regions. Indeed, the permanent substitution of chemical fertilizers for organic ones lessens the organic matter restored to the soil.

Excerpted from: *Fleury, A. and Mollard, A. "Agriculture, système social et environnement" ("Farming, Social System and Environment") IREP—CNEEJA, Grenoble, July 1976, p. 327.*

Energy Limitations of Farming in Industrialized Countries

Today's underdeveloped countries have a legitimate ambition to modernize their farming. However, they often try to do it by following the Western example, which because of structural, economic, and human handicaps may result in failure. Furthermore, if the estimate of the energy that is consumed by American farmers is accurate, spreading the American system would result in a demand for four billion barrels of oil each year to feed humanity (Fevrier and Poly, 1979).

Excerpted from: *Fevrier, R. and Poly, J. "Évolution prévisible du monde rural et du secteur agro-alimentaire" ("Foreseeable Evolution of the Rural World and the Food Production and Processing Sector") Note pour la 4th Conférence de Travail des Directeurs de la Recherche Agronomique, OCDE, Paris, nov 1979.*

Disrupting the Natural Balance

When an insecticide is sprayed on a designated surface, a significant amount of toxic substance is carried far away by air currents no matter what distribution method is used. As a result, insecticide residues have now spread throughout the entire world (Dajoz, 1969). This can be compared to radioactive fallout that results from nuclear testing (Woodwell, 1967). An aerial application of DDT on a New Brunswick forest at a ratio of 4.4 kilograms per hectare during a period of seven years showed that half the product used was dispersed in the atmosphere by the wind; the rest could be found three years after the last treatment at a concentration of 5.6 kilograms per hectare in the soil's deep mineral stratum.

A large number of analyses have been made of DDT residue because this insecticide has been used extensively for a long time, shows up easily, and persists for many years due to its great stability. It is estimated that it takes about ten years for half the accumulated DDT, no matter where it is, to disintegrate. Twenty years after a coastal swamp of the United States was sprayed with DDT to destroy mosquito larvae, Woodwell found 35 kilograms per hectare of DDT in the outer layers of mud.

The following examples show the extent to which the presence of DDT has become universal. This insecticide has been found in trout of New Zealand in a concentration of 0.6 to 0.8 parts per million (ppm); in Adelia penguins of Antarctica in a concentration of 0.015 to 0.18 ppm, and in seals of the same region in a similar concentration; in birds, shellfish, and plankton in the United States in a concentration varying from 0.41 to 138 ppm depending on the species; in dolphins in Florida in a concentration of 220 ppm; and finally in grebes, fish-eating birds, in a concentration of 1,600 ppm in California. DDT has been found in human fatty tissue (where it is soluble and accumulates readily) in the United States, Canada, Great Britain, France, Hungary, Israel, and India in concentrations varying from 2.2 to 31 ppm, depending on the region.

This list includes regions, such as the Antarctic, where insecticides have never been used and where DDT could only have gotten there by sea or air currents or by way of poisoned migrant animals. DDT has also been found in fish living in the open sea, in subterranean levels of water, and in most large American rivers.

Insecticides constitute a grave danger, since they accumulate little by little along the food chain: DDT is found in a concentration of 0.04 ppm in freshwater plankton; fish that eat plankton contain DDT in a concentration of 1 ppm; seagulls that feed on fish have up to 75 ppm of the insecticide in their tissues. In other words, carnivorous animals at the top of the food chain can concentrate more than a thousand times the amount of toxic substances in their bodies.

An example of this was given by Hunt and Bischoff. A California lake was treated with DDT at a level of 0.014 ppm to destroy mosquito larvae. The DDT concentrated in the plankton (5 ppm), then passed into plankton-eating fish (40 to 1,000 ppm), then carnivorous fish (350 to 2,500 ppm). This caused a high mortality rate in fish-eating birds, reducing the number of reproducing pairs at the lake from 1,000 to 30.

Upsetting nature's balance with insecticides has unknown consequences that can unleash a rapid multiplying of pests whose spread needs to be checked. In this area, unfortunately, we do not lack examples. The following is one case:

Habrochila ghesquieri is a flat insect parasite of the coffee shrub common to the eastern part of the Belgian Congo and to Uganda. It often causes considerable damage to plantations. To get rid of the parasite, many plantation owners have resorted to massive sprayings of DDT-based products. The result has been exactly the opposite of what they had hoped. The *Habrochila* is multiplying in every plot of land treated, causing much more serious, sometimes catastrophic, damage.

Extensive research has been carried out, establishing that:

1. *Habrochila* is virtually immune to DDT.
2. Another insect, *Apollodotus chinai*, a carnivore, actively preys on *Habrochila*, its chief source of food; *Apollodotus* consumes 10 to 15 *Habrochila* daily and has shown itself to be extremely vulnerable to DDT. The insecticide, therefore, destroyed the carnivorous species without reducing the plant-eating species. Rid of its natural predator, *Habrochila* has thus been able to multiply unchecked.

Excerpted from: *Dajoz, R. "Les insecticides" ("Insecticides")*
Presses Universitaires de France, Collection "Que sais-je?" no. 829,
Paris, 1969, p. 128.

Harmful Effects
of Chemical Pesticides

The harmful effects of pesticides appear slowly. Chemical treatments cause rapid multiplication of pests other than those specifically treated: successive generations of these pests—generations which are resistant to insecticides—become more numerous from year to year. Massive and repeated insecticide use has finally made us familiar with these disadvantages, but it has taken a long time.

These compounds are quite toxic to humans and other vertebrates, so users must take many precautions. In France, as in most other countries, regulatory boards require a precise determination of immediate effects, possible consequences, and chronic aspects of chemical pesticides. Particular attention is paid to their role in causing cancer and birth defects.

As new pesticides are developed, they should be studied to understand what soil residues and metabolites they might form. This can help reduce the risk to microorganisms that aid in the decomposition of the soil's organic matter.

To satisfy these requirements, large companies perform long and costly experiments on many different animals. As a result, any toxic reaction to these products in human beings must be due to ignorance of normal, recommended use. Nevertheless, bird populations, in particular, are exposed repeatedly to the dangers of many pesticides. Ramade (1974) recalls the great slaughter of sparrows caused by DDT treatments to eradicate the bark beetle on elm trees in the United States.

The concentration in trophic chains is now a well-established phenomenon. For example, cultivated plants, such as the carrot, concentrate the heptachlorine present in the treated soil, and thus become a source of pollution for animals that eat them. These animals are themselves the prey of other predators. Accordingly, the amount of residues is less in plants than in omnivores, becoming greater in predators, notably the sparrow hawk which feeds on other birds and insects (Ramade, 1974).

Because of their low numbers, their low rate of reproduction, and their position at the end of trophic chains, birds of prey are particularly susceptible to this chain of events. The effect of organochlorine residues on their reproduction has been demonstrated: delay in egg laying, reduced number of eggs (bordering on sterility in females), abnormal shell fragility as a reduction in estrogens inhibits proper calcification, and high embryo and chick mortality. The biology of earthworms also figures prominently in this process. Except for certain fungicides like benlate, earthworms are resistant to most pesticides and can accumulate them in their bodies without consequence; but woe to the birds (woodcocks, blackbirds, etc.) who eat these worms! The multiplication of the pests that are not treated with chemicals is another serious disadvantage. An important example can be seen in the cultivation of cotton in the Americas:

Over a ten-year period, the desire to curtail the boll weevil *Anthonomus grandis* necessitated treating plants with methyl and ethyl parathion, up to 30 or 40 times per growth cycle. However, these chemical treatments eventually resulted in an impasse for cotton growers in North and Central America: severe attacks by the moths *Heliothis zea*, *Trichoplusia ni*, and *Spodoptera exiqua*; by *Aphis gossypii*; and by tetranychids resulted, forcing plantation owners to raise other crops. In northeastern Mexico the cotton crop shrank from 300,000 hectares in the 1950s to 500 hectares 20 years later.

Two phenomena brought this about: first, changes in the chemical composition and metabolism of treated plants made them more favorable to certain species, especially acarids and cochineals, which began multiplying at a much faster rate (Chaboussou, 1980). Second, the entire complex of natural enemies controlling the population levels of insects and acarids was destroyed. These insect-eating parasites and predators are often more vulnerable to insecticides than the target pests.

Studies on the evolution of the plant-eating acarid populations *Panonychus ulmi* and *Tetranychus viennensis*, conducted for almost ten years by M. Perrier in apple orchards in Versailles and in Sarthe, have clearly demonstrated the existence of more than 17 auxiliary species (Heteropteres and acaridan predator species) of parasites and predators which help control acaridan populations naturally if pesticides are not used.

We are also seeing resistant generations of many crop-destroying insects and mites more frequently. The amount of an effective substance must therefore be increased each year, which means increases in cost of operation, risk of toxicity and residue, and effects on the bioecology. Often the substance becomes practically useless, once the pests have developed an immunity to it.

12   *Hunger and Health*

As a general rule, this resistance is not developed against a single product, but rather takes in all derivatives of the same chemical origin. The genetic workings of natural selection proceed at a pace determined by the insect's fertility and annual number of generations, as well as by the type of compound. This phenomenon occurred within one year with the mosquito *Anopheles gambiae* using dieldrin, and within ten years with the moth *Spodoptera ittoralis* using organophosphorated compounds (Brown, 1974).

Because of the worldwide importance of this phenomenon, the Food and Agriculture Organization (FAO) has organized a group of experts who meet periodically to examine the list of resistant species, define viable methods of control through evaluation of this resistance, and propose solutions where crop protection is known to have failed.

In 1967, this group inventoried about 250 resistant species, including 100 resistant to DDT, 150 to organochlorine, 60 to organophosphorated compounds, and more than 10 to carbamates. Some species showed a resistance to several types of pesticides: 40 percent of the cases involved Diptera; 15 percent, Lepidoptera; 15 percent, Hemiptera; and 10 percent, Acaridans.

Because of this phenomenon, there is increasing difficulty in protecting important crops—such as rice in Japan, cotton in North and South America and the Near East, and even cattle in Australia—from mosquitoes. In the southern Tyrol, the pear sucker has developed resistance to all known insecticides, forcing tree growers to uproot 7,000 hectares of trees. There is also cause for concern in grain storage. Malathion, which has been used against insects up to now, is becoming less and less effective in many regions. In spite of their still limited number, cases of pest resistant to fumigants constitute a very serious threat to world food production and consumption (FAO, 1973).

It should be noted that very little success can be expected with renewed use of these pesticides, even after a long hiatus. It is therefore necessary to turn to organic methods of dealing with this problem, a problem often aggravated by the abuse of chemicals.

Excerpted from: *"Aspect écologique des problèmes phytosanitaires" ("Ecological Aspect of Phystosanitary Problems")* Purpan, *no. 99, April-May-June 1976; 272 av. de Grande-Bretagne, 31076 Toulouse Cedex.*

The Growing Resistance of Insects to Pesticides

As part of the preparation of the Monograph on Resistance, G. P. Georghiou and H. T. Reynolds have compiled and computerized the results of the third world survey for resistance. The first world survey in 1965 reported 182 pests as having developed some degree of resistance to one or more pesticides. The list in the 1968 survey included 228 species. The present survey which includes all species of Acarina and Insecta found to be resistant totals 364, of which 304 of the cases have been confirmed by laboratory tests. However, it should be noted that this list includes cases of resistance in Culicidae (83 species) which had not been included in the earlier surveys. Thus, the total number of resistant species (minus the Culicidae) now stands at 281.

It was noted that, in the ten-year period, 1965–1975, the list of resistant species on cotton grew from 20 to 33. The relative increase in numbers of species reported to be resistant on rice was similar, having increased from 8 to 14 in the ten-year interval. This general increase in numbers of resistant species has possibly also occurred on other crops that receive repeated applications of insecticides. The increasing number of species reported to have developed resistance is of serious concern. However, the intensification of resistance problems is cause for even greater concern. The increases in importance are due both to loss in effectiveness of more types of insecticides and to geographical extension, as more and more regions report resistance.

The situation regarding resistance in plant pathogens is a particular cause for concern. Very few reports of resistance in plant pathogens were received in 1965. Since the development and intensive use of the systemic fungicides in recent years, reports of resistance have increased drastically. At the present time, more than 67 species of plant pathogen have developed resistance to one or more of 42 chemicals. A large percentage of these involve resistance to systemic fungicides, especially benzimidazoles.

Excerpted from: *"Monograph on Resistance of Agricultural Pests,"* *FAO report, Washington, D.C., 1976, pp. 9-10.*

The Cost of Pesticides

It is interesting to examine the relative costs of pesticide research and development. In 1972, it was estimated that, in the United States, one new pesticide emerged for every 10,000 compounds tested, that the time from discovery to market is eight to ten years, and that the cost for all this is in excess of $10 million (WHO, 1976). This figure would undoubtedly be significantly higher now.

It is also reasonable to assume that additional safety requirements for pesticides will become mandatory in many countries. These may include two-year cancer studies on laboratory animals; mutation and birth defect studies; toxic effects on primates; and perhaps human metabolic studies as well. These additional tests might increase the cost of the safety testing to over $1 million per compound.

Excerpted from: *OMS (Organisation Mondiale de la Santé) (World Health Organization Technical Report Series) "Risques pour la santé liés aux nouveaux polluants de l'environnement" ("Health Hazards from New Environmental Pollutants") no. 586, OMS, Genève, 1976.*

Agricultural Methods and Soil Fertility

We should make a few remarks on methods of soil conservation and soil fertility.

One of the biggest differences between the ecology of temperate zones and tropical zones is soil fertility. Ferric soils, often deficient in phosphorus, calcium, and magnesium, are low in their ability to exchange cations. Their fertility depends on a very high decomposition rate of organic matter to form humus. This necessitates, as a base for fertility, a diet permanently enriched with organic matter. All the methods noted in the preceding pages have the single goal of promoting organic recycling. To complete this strategy, complementary measures for the treatment of organic matter, application of mineral fertilizers, and corresponding mechanical equipment are needed.

It is the compost heap that first provides this indispensable way of maintaining fertility. Although this method is understood everywhere, it is rarely implemented in a systematic manner. Manure, mixed with a lot of plant matter from the surrounding area, guarantees a high-quality product the following season.

Excerpted from: *Egger, Dr. K. E. "Vers l'agroécologie optimale— Étude de la conservation des sols dans quelques ORD en Haute Volta" ("Toward Optimal Agroecology—Study of Soil Conservation in Some ORD in Upper Volta") Polycopié—Ouagadougou/Heidelberg, February 1980, p. 60.*

Composting in West Africa

To illustrate composting techniques, here are three observations made by practitioners in West Africa: Father Terrible, a missionary at the Kossoghen seminary in Upper Volta, had his students try composting. They used the ditch composting method, used and developed by Howard in India (Howard, 1947). The primary matter was brush herbs and a little dung when available. The cut-up herbs and dung were put into a ditch during the dry season and then left there during the entire rainy season and the following dry season. It was a long period of composting (more than one year). Perhaps this is not agronomically ideal, but because of the rains, the pile did not require watering.

When this compost was applied to crops, the results were remarkable: crop production was about two times higher on composted plots than on plots with chemical fertilizer and two to five times higher than the neighbor's plots which had no added fertilizer. Scientists will say that this experiment is not valid because there was not any repetition of treatments nor was it done with scientific strictness. For this reason it is necessary to repeat this type of experiment under rigorous conditions in different developing countries.

A similar observation was made by a rural farmer whom I met one day in a remote village in Mali. He had read an article on the composting of brushwood and tried to do it himself. Here again, he did not follow any precise measures, but he observed a considerable increase in crop yields and a longer fruit-bearing season.

Another interesting example is that of a farmer in Upper Volta. He was a sedentary *Peulh* (a stock-breeder by trade who'd become a farmer); owning livestock, he did not lack manure. After following the advice of local farmers (sowing in lines, using selected varieties and complete fertilizers), he noticed little increase in his yield and none at all in his income; he stopped using the fertilizers and began burying straw and using manure regularly. His yield is now two to three times higher than that of his neighbors.

Today's research centers give the same results as the above examples using much more scientific methods. As an example, here are the conclusions of an 18-year experiment carried out at the Saria research center, Upper Volta:

> *Mineral fertilizer alone, especially when used in large amounts, caused a lowering of the soil's fertility, especially its pH, affecting the exchangeable bases. When soil acidification is high it leads to nutrient problems (blocking of certain elements).*
>
> *Used in small amounts, dung helps the soil maintain certain physico-chemical characteristics (pH). Used in large amounts, it improves them.*
>
> *It would be beneficial to coordinate the raising of livestock and farming, and to increase crop recycling using organic processes (aerobic/anaerobic composting) that can prevent the formation of toxic substances.**

**Source: M. R. Sedogo, J. Pichot, J. F. Poulain, "Évolution de la fertilité d'un sol ferrugineux tropical sous l'influence de fumures minérales et organiques" ("Evolution of the Fertility of Ferruginous Tropical Soil under the Influence of Mineral and Organic Fertilizers") IRAT, Station de Saria, Republic of Upper Volta, October 1979.*

It is interesting to note that a report published by an official center in Upper Volta, *Institut de Recherches Agronomiques Tropicales et des Cultures Vivrières (IRAT)*, concluded that composting has many benefits. Results from the experiments the research center carried out on composting (anaerobic and aerobic methods) and sorghum production appear in table 1–2.

These figures show the superiority of aerobic composting to other organic methods. They also demonstrate, according to chemists, the benefits of mineral nitrogen supplies. It is true that under the conditions of this experiment, mineral nitrogen brought noticeably greater yields, since the soil was poor in nitrogen and organic matter and the rotation crop included very few, if any, legumes.

But the practice of balanced crop rotation and associated crops would no doubt permit equivalent yield without mineral nitrogen. Experiments should be done using these methods, because the general use of mineral nitrogen, even in amounts as low as 60 kilograms per hectare, is impossible in many parts of the developing world, primarily for economic reasons. If 2.5 million hectares of cultivated land in Upper Volta received 60 kilograms of nitrogen per hectare in the form of nitrate fertilizers, this would represent 150,000 tons of nitrogen, a consumption of 300,000 tons of petroleum. This figure is three times greater than the total consumption of petroleum products in Upper Volta and represents an expense of about 35 billion francs, CFA, which is a 50 percent increase in the country's total imports.

Table 1-2   Sorghum production (Grain E 35–1) in kilograms per hectare

Soil improvement method	Without nitrogen	With nitrogen (60 kg/ha)
Control	1,831	2,796
Straw (10 t/ha)	1,652	3,427
Manure (10 t/ha)	2,409	3,591
Aerobic compost (10 t/ha)	2,505	3,688
Anaerobic compost (10 t/ha)	2,304	3,601

Source: IRAT/Haute-Volta, Extrait du rapport de synthèse 1980, Partie B1: Agronomie, mars 1981.

Excerpted from: *Aubert, C. "Quelle politique agro-alimentaire pour le Tiers-Monde?"* (*"What Agro-Alimentary Policies for the Third World?"*) Nature et Progrès, *no. 76, Paris, September-October 1982.*

Burying Surplus Harvest in Senegal

Manure and crop residues form the basis of organic fertilizers. The benefits of recycling them are illustrated by an experiment with peanut crops carried out at the Center for Agronomic Research at Bambey, Senegal.

Table 1-3

Farming method	Water reserves 1 month after planting (mm)	Peanut yield (q/ha)
Burned fallow land	21	10
Buried fallow land	64	18
Millet with buried leaves	79	20

Excerpted from: *Aubert, C.* L'agriculture biologique—Pourquoi et comment la pratiquer (Organic Farming—Why and How to Practice It) *Éd. Le Courrier du Livre, Paris, 1977, p. 363.*

Agricultural Methods to Supplement Composting

The practice of mulching should be used in conjunction with compost applications whenever possible. As the mulch decomposes, soil microorganisms will reinforce nitrogen assimilation. Mulches made of rice straw or dried brush help in the control of weeds and reduce evaporation of moisture from the soil, providing protection against water shortages during the growing season.

Aside from classic NPK fertilizers, which can play an auxiliary role when first applied to depleted soil, it is necessary to plan a program that uses mineral fertilizers based on the resources available. For example, in Upper Volta there are three possible sources of mineral fertilizer available:

1. Natural phosphates
2. Calcareous or dolomitic rocks
3. Basic siliceous rocks.

However, their value and effectiveness are closely related to very high bacterial activity in the soil which occurs only when a great amount of organic matter has been previously added.

Excerpted from: *Egger, Dr. K. E. "Vers l'agroécologie optimale—Étude de la conservation des sols dans quelques ORD en Haute Volta" ("Toward Optimal Agroecology—Study of Soil Conservation in Some ORD in Upper Volta") Polycopié—Ouagadougou/Heidelberg, February 1980, p. 60.*

Advantages of Intercropping

By looking at the ways different authors emphasize the advantages of mixed cropping, it is possible to examine their validity on a technical level (Bergeret, 1977). A list of observations and advantages follows:

- Intercropping species makes excellent use of environmental factors—water, nutritive elements, sunlight, optimal spatial and temporal combinations of leaf and root organs—thereby meeting nutrient needs and conserving topsoil. Erosion and leaching are reduced. Complementary aspects can be reinforced by synergistic relationships such as symbiosis.
- Insect attacks and diseases, while more varied, tend to be reduced. Also, weed populations may be kept in check. The variety of crops brings a distribution of risks, since all plants are not affected to the same degree by climatic and ecological hazards. This provides genuine security for the farmer.
- Field work is evenly distributed throughout the year, and the work is more productive in general.
- Increased production and yields lead to greater income, resulting from the effects of synergy.

An example of these advantages comes from Nigeria where comparisons between associated crop and single crop cultivation were made on two levels: under primitive conditions and under improved conditions (mineral fertilizer, better varieties).

Under the primitive conditions, there was a variety of crop associations, with a preference for a millet/sorghum combination. In monetary terms, associated crops surpassed the single crops by 62 percent.

Under improved conditions, the best sorghum/cowpea combination showed surplus revenues of more than 60 percent for the entire cultivated area when compared with sorghum cultivated alone. For crops planted in alternating rows (late sorghum plus one combination of two successive crops), larger profits were shown than with late sorghum as a single crop. This profit was double in monetary value at relatively high yield levels (two tons per hectare) for the single crop sorghum.

The best combination tested (two rows of early millet plus cowpea, one row of late dwarf sorghum) showed the following advantages and disadvantages:

● The loss of millet production in relation to single crop millet was minimal, less than 10 percent.
● The income per entire cultivated area was higher and work hours were more even.
● Risks from erosion and drought were minimized.
● The mechanization of most sowing operations was possible using the best combinations (sowing by tractor!).

The only disadvantages noted were certain harvest and sowing difficulties under humid conditions and the need for good drying conditions after millet and corn harvests. These disadvantages, being easily remedied, clearly tip the balance in favor of associated crops whether it be with improved crops or not.

Excerpted from: *Bergeret, A. "Vers une plus large autonomie alimentaire du Tiers-Monde" ("Toward Greater Food System Autonomy in the Third World") doctoral thesis, University of Paris I, June 1977.*

Leguminous Plants Associated with Maize (Cover Crop)

Grain-maize is the main crop at the bottom of the Cochabamba valley. Normally no other crop is planted after the harvest. The few weeds are grazed by the animals and the soil remains exposed to the sun and wind until the next rainy season: erosion is inevitable.

Trials with leguminous plants under cover have been carried out on maize, in order to devise a method of maintaining plant cover during the winter, in accordance with the principles of organic farming, while at the same time ensuring improved soil structure and increased humus content, as well as forage production.

The use of leguminous plants under cover is a specific form of associated cropping. Once the maize has reached a level of 25 centimeters, clover is sown after mechanical hoeing to control weeds. The maize can develop to the full, while by the time it is ripe the clover will only have reached a height of some 30 centimeters which enables it to stifle the weeds without in any way competing with the maize. Harvesting the maize removes competition for water, light, and nutrients, so that the clover can now develop rapidly and become an economic forage crop without the necessity of recultivating the soil.

Fourteen varieties of leguminous plants were tested in order to see which plant would be most suitable as a cover crop, taking into account the local conditions. Here we tried not only to discover the best adapted plant, but also to establish the optimum sowing date (in relation to the stage of development of the maize), as well as the simplest sowing technique to be adopted in small and medium farms.

Table 1–4 clearly shows that *Vicia villosa* is the best associated plant in the trial conditions. It ensured the highest grain-maize yields, with the exception of maize grown with *Onobrychis vicifolia*. However, taking into account the yield of green forage during August—a period when forage is usually in short supply—*V. villosa* is far superior to the 13 other leguminous plants for use as a cover crop.

In terms of sowing date, we found that the best *forage yields* were obtained when maize and *Vicia villosa* were sown at the same time (36 tons per hectare). However, compared with sowing the leguminous plant immediately after hoeing, the method resulted in a slight competition with the maize (0.3 tons per hectare). The ideal method, therefore, consists of sowing *V. villosa* (40 kilograms per hectare) immediately after weed control.

On a trial plot on poor nonfertilized soil in a campesino's field, *Vicia villosa* ensured increased yields of the grain-maize Uchuquilla (old local variety) and Choclero 2 (improved variety). With another new variety of grain-maize—Aychasara—which apparently does not require any special manuring, yields were good in the absence of *V. villosa*; in its presence, however, the competition with this maize variety was such, that yields fell by half compared with those obtained without *V. villosa*.

Results of this kind show clearly that when growing leguminous plants in this way, what is important is not only the leguminous plant species, variety, or sowing date, but also the variety chosen for the main crop.

Table 1-4	14 different plants sown as cover crops in association with maize *Pairumani test, 1979–1980 (alt. 2,620 m)*		
	Yield in grain maize[1] (t/ha)	Forage yield, 2d cutting (GM/t/ha[2])	Percentage of soil cover by the associated plant (excluding weeds)
Medicago lupulina	6.35	9.00	47
Medicago sativa	7.47	10.24	31
Lotus corniculatus	6.63	3.67	3
Trifolium pratense	6.49	10.40	40
Trifolium repens	5.74	7.23	37
Trifolium resupinatum	6.26	4.60	13
Trifolium alexandreium	6.18	9.87	23
Trifolium subterraneum	7.10	4.03	24
Trifolium hybridum	7.12	5.10	4
Helilotus albus	7.72	5.97	46
Anthyllis vulneraria	7.03	5.63	3
Onobrychis vicifolia	9.66	4.20	3
Vicia sativa	5.36	15.62[3]	23
Vicia villosa	8.70	20.43	61
No association	5.67	2.00	42[4]
SSD[5] (P ≤ 0.05)	**2.90**	**3.60**	**19**

1 Maize variety: Composite 13
2 GM: green matter
3 First cutting only
4 Weeds only
5 Smallest significant difference

Excerpted from: *Annual report, Cochabamba Agrobiology Project, F. Augstburger, 1981, Swiss Foundation for the Promotion of Biological Agriculture, Oberwill/BL, Simon I. Patino and Pro Bolivia Foundations, Geneva.*

Maintaining Low-Cost Soil Fertility

Maintaining the amount of humus in farming soil should be a primary concern to farmers because humus guarantees the soil's continuing capacity to produce nutritious food crops. Some primitive means still in use to maintain humus should be studied and more widely popularized. For example, the Mexican horticulturists who cultivate the Chinampas ("swamp gardens") on Lake Xochimilco near Mexico City use fertilization techniques that have proven their worth for 20 centuries. These gardeners use aquatic plants, which are abundant along the lake's edge, as well as mud that is rich in organic residue, and bat droppings from nearby calcareous caves. In addition, the use of cow or horse manure has filled out the range of their fertilization methods.

Numerous farmers and gardeners throughout the world use classical methods that should also be made better known so others could apply them. The Wollaytas farmers of southwest Ethiopia widely use the technique of mulching; in Southeast Asia azolla cultivated in rice fields is an excellent green fertilizer; in France, different experiments were carried out with compost preparations based on brushwood, all with the same goal: to use organic material to the fullest.

Through research efforts, "new" methods of resource-efficient farming are also being developed (Collombon, 1980). In India, the International Agricultural Research Institute of New Delhi focused on a simple cultivation method for blue-green algae at 10 kilograms per hectare which resulted in a 15 percent increase in rice production. The method used involved judiciously combining an alga already known locally with a modern fertilizer source: superphosphate. The chief feature of this technique, besides its low cost (7 rupees versus 100 rupees for providing an equivalent amount of nitrogen per hectare), was the fact that the farmer himself produced this biological fertilizer. All that was needed was a ditch made watertight with a plastic cover to which was added earth treated with 200 grams of superphosphate of ammonia.

Indian researchers have found an alternative to the regular price increases in chemical fertilizer, thereby making fertilizers accessible to the large majority of small farmers. Moreover, the Indians hypothesize that production cost of the fertilizing algae will become negligible when the algae become acclimated to the medium and begin to reproduce spontaneously.

Excerpted from: *Collombon, J. M. "Demain une agriculture plus écologique—Prémisses et promesses" ("Tomorrow, a More Ecological Agriculture—Premises and Promises") Polycopié, June 1980, p. 16.*

Direct Use of Natural Phosphates

Various studies have shown that phosphorus deficiency is the most serious limiting factor in farm production in almost all of the countries of West Africa. We do not claim to have a solution to this problem. We simply want to draw attention to the results of some French tropical agronomic researchers, showing that many countries in Africa could draw phosphates directly from their natural resources and avoid having to import soluble phosphates. Numerous African countries have resources rich in natural phosphates. The phosphate beds at Thies in Senegal, Tilemsi in Mali, Arli in Upper Volta, Ahoua in Nigeria, and Anecho in Togo are well known—to name just those in French-speaking Africa.

The recent tripling of the price of phosphates on the world market gives considerable importance to the possibility of using local phosphates. But to be economically advantageous, these phosphates must be obtainable with a minimum of industrial processing. The only indispensable operation is the pulverization (the fineness of grind is very important for the assimilation of low-solubility phosphates). Small-scale equipment is quite sufficient to carry out this operation.

Supported by research done since 1967, the *Institut de Recherches Agronomiques Tropicales et des Cultures Vivrières (IRAT)* has observed the effectiveness of natural phosphates, whatever their composition. Several examples demonstrate this:

• Comparisons between natural phosphates and soluble phosphates show that the best way to improve crop yields as well as the soil's balance of phosphoric acid and lime consists in using natural phosphates buried with green manure at the beginning of the rotation. The use of phosphates in Thies, Senegal, whether as annual fertilizer or basal dressing, always enriches the soil with assimilable phosphorus.

• In Nigeria, experiments on three types of dune soil more or less deficient in phosphate led to the conclusion that a correction can be made by a basal dressing of 400 to 500 kilograms of phosphate fertilizer per hectare for highly depleted soil and 150 to 300 kilograms per hectare for moderately depleted soil. Under these conditions there is improvement even the first year.

• Testing done in Upper Volta showed that ground natural phosphates are effective for sorghum during the first year of use. Although their effect in this instance was inferior to that of soluble phosphate, it did bring crop yield increases, some as much as 100 percent. When used for several years with phosphate-based fertilizers at the beginning of the rotation, ground natural phosphates were practically equivalent to soluble phosphates.

• In Mali, the response of dry crops (grains and peanuts, in particular) to phosphate from Tilemsi was excellent the first year. And a delayed reaction, three years after its application, is still being observed. In rotation, a high degree of effectiveness was observed with a phosphate-based fertilizer from Tilemsi at 450 to 600 kilograms of phosphate per hectare. The latter amount results in crop yields as high as those with an annual application of a soluble phosphate. Finally, the effectiveness of natural phosphate has been verified in most of Mali, even in zones with little rainfall.

• In fertilization and maintenance of corn/peanut rotation, Togo's phosphate had no effect the first year but brought substantial crop increases over the next three years.

The use of natural phosphates has already been popularized in certain countries. The IRAT thinks that technical bases are now solid, and that economic studies, taking into account the cost of extraction, pulverizing, and distribution, would show that these phosphates can, in most cases with a minimum of rainfall and some soil acidity (the normal state for most African soils), replace imported phosphate fertilizers.

Excerpted from: *"Fertiliser naturellement"* *("Fertilizing Naturally")* Cérès, *March-April 1976.*

Sources of Fertilizer in the Third World

As seen in table 1–5, most developing countries are wasting their natural fertilizer resources and supplementing crops primarily with imported or factory-produced fertilizers.

Table 1-5	Amounts of natural fertilizing elements, whether used or not, available in the Third World in 1971, compared to amounts of chemical fertilizers that the Third World produced, imported, and consumed during the same year (millions of tons)

	Nitrogen fertilizers N	Phosphate fertilizers P	Potassium fertilizers K	Total NPK
Animal wastes	17.80	4.91	14.12	36.83
Farm compost	9.54	3.34	9.54	22.42
Human wastes	12.25	2.87	2.61	17.73
Urban sewers	1.43	0.29	0.86	2.58
Urban compost	0.48	0.38	0.57	1.43
Miscellaneous	6.63	4.44	11.35	22.42
Available organic elements	48.13	16.23	39.05	103.41
Chemical fertilizers produced	3.28	1.65	0.30	5.23
Chemical fertilizers consumed	5.87	2.61	1.44	9.93

Excerpted from: *"Fertiliser naturellement"* (*"Fertilizing Naturally"*) Cérès, *March-April 1976.*

Comparing Organic and Conventional Farming in the United States

The commercial-scale organic farmers in our studies made little use of methods that most farmers would regard as exotic; rather, as alternatives to chemical fertilization and pest-control methods they used rotations with legume forages and other practices similar to those found on many Corn Belt farms, but relied more heavily on these techniques than did conventional farmers. Because of the heavier reliance on legume forage as a nitrogen source, organic farmers may not be able to choose an exclusively cash-grain operation, whereas, for better or worse, conventional farmers have this choice.

Slightly lower gross production per unit of cropland on the organic farms was largely offset by comparable reductions in operating expenses, so that crop production was about equally profitable on the two types of farms except in a year that had extremely favorable weather. The exact comparison appears to depend on growing conditions, with the organic farms doing relatively better under the abnormally poor conditions of the mid-1970s, but relatively poorer when conditions improved in 1978. Except for wheat, a minor crop in the Corn Belt for which organic farms had much poorer yields, yields of most organically raised crops generally ranged from about the same to about 10 percent lower than on the conventional farms.

Excerpted from: *Lockeretz, W. et al. "Organic Farming in the Corn Belt"* Science, *vol. 211, February 1981, pp. 540-47.*

Effect of Fertilizers and Pesticides on Disease Resistance of Plants

Fertilization and pesticides condition plant resistance (Chaboussou, 1974). It is necessary to understand that different products used in chemical pest control—whether mineral or organic, fungicides, acaricides or insecticides—are susceptible to penetrating the plant under certain conditions and therefore of acting on its metabolism.

These pesticides may saturate the plant with metal or metalloid compounds which contain copper, iron, zinc, manganese, sulfur, phosphorus, etc. Following this saturation they can either stimulate or inhibit metabolic activity. Such effects depend not only on the type of product and the amount used, but also on when it was used and the plant's initial condition. Thus, pesticides, specifically organic ones, can act hormonally on the plant's chief physiological processes: respiration, transpiration, photosynthesis.

It is generally agreed that a plant's resistance develops primarily from biochemical factors, not strictly physical ones. According to our understanding of trophobiosis (Chaboussou,

1967): "All vital processes find themselves rigidly dependent upon the satisfaction of the nutritional needs of the living organism, whether plant or animal." In other words: the plant will be attacked in the measure that its biochemical state corresponds to the trophic demands of the parasite in question.

Therefore, it is important to emphasize the role that soluble substances (amino acids, reducible glucosides) play in the susceptibility of a plant to its various predators. These compounds appear to affect the plant's attractiveness to mites or insects as well as its susceptibility to disease.

Chart 1

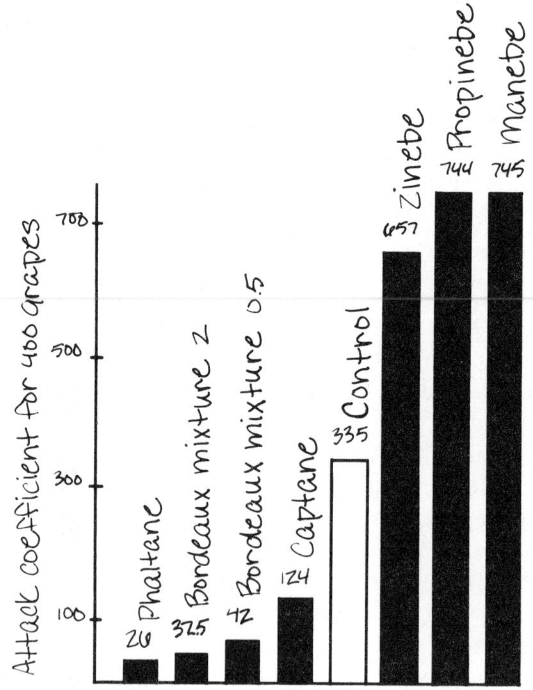

The attack coefficient of powdery mildew is two times higher for the vine treated with zinebe, propinebe, and manebe than for the control vine (La Tresne trial, 1966, Cabernet-Sauvignon Vine Variety, four repetitions).

For example, Hoffman and Samish (1969) have shown that amino acids accumulate in the tissues of citrus plants each time available potassium is insufficient or excessive. However, an adequate cationic balance does not appear sufficient *alone* to insure that the plant's metabolism will allow for optimal proteogenesis and, therefore, resistance. The plant must have the energy necessary to carry out the proteogenesis from the materials that are assimilated through nutrition. This, it seems, is the role of growth materials which can come from organic fertilizers (humic acids, indolacetic acid).

Thus, the combined action of manure and mineral fertilizers appears to explain the results obtained by Mehani (1969) in regard to the degeneration of the artichoke "Violet de Provence" as noted in Tunisia (chart 2). His results may help explain the beneficial action of humus, often empirically noted by farmers in regard to disease incidence.

Chart 2

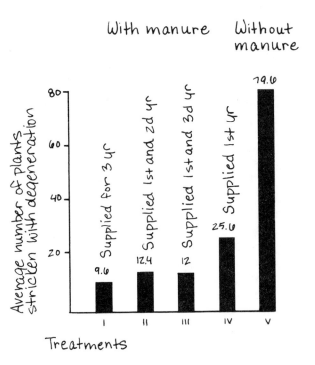

It seems that the effect of a pesticide on a plant's physiology can be controlled by using a judicious balance of organic and mineral fertilizers. It is therefore up to the farmer to know how to use these extrinsic factors in conjunction with the plant's genetic potential in order to assure the plant's health and protection.

Excerpted from: Chaboussou, F. *"Fumures, traitements et autres facteurs extrinsèques conditionnent la résistance de la plante"* *("Fertilizers, Treatments, and Other Extrinsic Factors Condition Plant Resistance")* Encyclopédie permanente d'agriculture biologique, Éd. Débard, Paris 1, Phytopathologie, Fumures, pp. 1-14, 1974.

Effect of Crop Associations on Yield and Parasite Attacks

As already discussed, crop associations (notably grains plus legumes) often promote greater yields while decreasing the number of parasite attacks.

It has been shown that planting methods that alter the ecology, such as crop associations, affect crop infestation because they affect the visual and olfactory reactions of species that invade crops (A. Brook, 1968; Raros, 1973; Dempster and Coaker, 1974).

Later, when crops are attacked by various species of parasites, the resultant insect preference for a crop will determine how much a particular species will damage the crop. In other words, certain crop associations can be used as diversion hosts, foils, or protectors.

Herrera and Harwood (1973) noted that in the association wheat/peanuts, infestation by wheat aphids (*Ostrinia furnicalis*) is less than for monoculture wheat, because the adult females are not attracted to the wheat when it is cultivated in association. Also, it is likely that a greater population of predator species raises the rate of destruction of aphid larvae. Herrera (1975) also showed that, although wide spaces between cultivated rows reduce boring insects, catch crops at high and low densities increase the effectiveness of predators, notably that of *Lycosa* species.

Traditional farmers in tropical countries have learned to take advantage of such cultivation systems to maintain a predator-prey balance. These traditional multiple cropping systems have not been equaled by modern agricultural technology because the long-term studies needed to understand them fully have not been carried out. To use crop associations efficiently in fighting parasites, it is first necessary to have a long-term management plan as well as a wise use of pesticides. In the past several years, we have tried to study the different aspects of the role that crop associations play in the control of parasites for the associations corn/cowpea and cassava/corn in different parts of Southwest Nigeria. In a series of experiments, some of which are still in progress, we evaluated the effects of corn/cowpea associations on the incidence of parasite species and their effect on the harvest yields of both crops. The results and observations of the 1975 experiments are summed up in table 1–6.

This table shows that with crop associations, the number of insecticide applications can be reduced to the rate of 400 grams of active substance per hectare instead of four to six applications (lindane/DDT are recommended) when cowpea is planted as a monoculture; this reduction is advantageous.

For the bushy variety, TVU 4557, the yield per hectare of cowpea as an associated crop in the same row is not significantly inferior to the cowpea as a monoculture. As a crop in alternate rows, cowpea yielded 800 kilograms hectare, which is substantially higher than the normal yield for the monoculture crop in southern Nigeria (Booker, 1964; Taylor, 1968).

With the semibushy variety, "Ife Brown," cowpea cultivated in association in the same row as the other species produced a yield superior to that of cowpea as either an alternate row crop or a monoculture. In addition, all these yields were considerably higher than average. The yield for corn in these experiments was 2,000 to 3,100 kilograms per hectare.

These results indicate that cowpea as a catch crop improves the yield of corn, probably because of both the nutritional compatibility between corn and nitrogen-fixing cowpea and a reduction of stem-boring insect infestation (Taylor, 1977).

Suryatna and Harwood (1976) showed that the association corn/peanut reduces the grain-boring insect populations by diminishing corn's predisposition to collect the eggs of boring insects and by increasing the rate of larvae mortality.

Table 1–6 also shows that the rate of damage caused by stem-boring insects is considerably higher for monoculture corn than for the two types of association. However, the factors responsible for this deviation are not yet clear.

Table 1-6 Yield comparisons of corn and cowpea planted as single crops and in two types of associations intended to combat parasites with minimal use of insecticides (kg/ha of dry grain)

Single or associated culture	Corn	Cowpea	Total grain yield per hectare	% total grain harvest loss to boring insects	% cowpea flower and pod loss due to maruca		% cowpea pod loss due to lasperyresia
					Flowers	Pods	
A. Corn alone	2,158.3 (c)	—	2,158.3	15.6 (a)	—	—	—
Corn + cowpea (crops in alternate rows)	2,666.6 (b)	000.0 (b)	3,466.6	10.2 (b)	18.8 (a)	16.4 (a)	17.3 (b)
Corn + cowpea (crops in same row)	3,091.6 (a)	1,200.0 (a)	4,291.6	8.5 (b)	10.3 (b)	17.5 (a)	24.0 (a)
Cowpea alone	—	1,250.0 (a)	1,250.0	—	15.2 (a)	18.6 (a)	13.3 (b)
B. Corn alone	2,631.0 (b)	—	2,631.0	16.2 (a)	—	—	—
Corn + cowpea (crops in alternate rows)	2,525.0 (c)	135.0 (b)	2,660.0	10.1 (b)	15.0 (a)	14.2 (b)	11.3 (a)
Corn + cowpea (crops in same row)	2,675.0 (a)	155.0 (a)	2,830.0	8.2 (b)	8.3 (b)	9.9 (c)	11.0 (a)
Cowpea alone	—	85.0 (c)	85.0	—	15.9 (a)	19.4 (a)	11.0 (a)

A. = cowpea variety TVU 4557

B. = cowpea variety "Ife Brown"

*Two applications of 0.1% monocrotophos in the amount of 400 g/ha of the active ingredient.

**The figures followed by the same letter are not significantly different from each other ($P=0.05$)

Excerpted from: *Taylor, T. A. "Les associations culturales, moyen de lutte contre les parasites des plantes en Afrique Tropicale" ("Crop Associations, Means of Struggle Against Plant Parasites in Tropical Africa")* Environnement Africain, *vol. II, November 1977, pp. 113-20.*

Associated Crop Trials: Potatoes, Beans, Lupines

A further example of the effect of associated crops on parasite attacks is shown in the test results with potatoes, beans, and lupines. Grade and storage life of potatoes are also indicated.

Table 1-7

	Potato leaves attacked by virus and cryptogram disease (%)	Potatoes in classes 1 & 2 (%)	Weight loss during storage[1] (%)
Potatoes (monoculture)	21	33	16
Lupines (monoculture)	—	—	—
Beans (monoculture)	—	—	—
Potatoes + lupines (cover crop)	10	41	10
Potatoes + beans (cover crop)	10	27	11
Potatoes + lupines (mixed crop)	16	31	9
Potatoes + beans (mixed crop)	12	20	10
SSD (P ≤ 0.05)[2]	7.6	9.3	NS

1 After 2 months in an ordinary cellar
2 SSD: Smallest significant difference

Excerpted from: *Annual report, Cochabamba Agrobiology Project,*
F. Augstburger, 1981, Swiss Foundation for the Promotion of Bio-
logical Agriculture, Oberwill/BL, Simon I. Patino and Pro Bolivia
Foundations, Geneva.

When Organic Methods Are the Best Weapon Against Pests

We can speak of organic plant protection when biological phenomena are consciously used to limit pests. More precisely, we define organic protection as the active reduction of sufficient numbers of pest species by using their natural enemies. Among these pests' enemies are higher animals (for example, insect-eating birds), predator or parasitic insects and mites, as well as consumers of undesirable plants and carriers of pest diseases.

Organic methods of plant protection present numerous ecological and economical advantages. Their use, however, poses some practical problems.

No species can multiply infinitely. It soon runs into obstacles, such as the high mortality that results from an increase in population density. Natural enemies are also part of this "breaking mechanism." The biological struggle is a tool that allows a balance to be established between the attacker and victim. It does not result in total extermination of the pest, thereby preserving the diversity of the environment.

Organic methods introduce no new elements; only that which already exists is used. But the action of natural enemies in repressing pests is often insufficient. For example, cultivating large areas of a certain plant sets up ideal conditions for the multiplication of plant-eating species. This is not the case for their enemies. The organic method, therefore, does more than just wait for nature's forces to regulate things. It demands an active intervention to counterbalance the upsetting of the natural balance caused by modern man with his high-yield farming and dense occupation.

The "useful" organisms can be manipulated thus:

1. by actively encouraging the species already available;
2. by introducing natural enemies belonging to the fauna of another part of the world, especially when the pest was introduced from the same spot;

3. by producing useful organisms on a large scale and by releasing them repeatedly.

In what follows, we will consider three forms of plant protection. Three groups of useful organisms are especially effective when released en masse: parasites, such as the Ichneumonides or nematodes; predators, such as mites or coccinella; and agents that cause disease in harmful insects, especially bacteria, fungi, protozoa (unicellular animals), and viruses.

Massive auxiliary releases of these and other species are often beneficial (even if associated with other methods), because they bring about a marked and relatively fast decrease in pests on the entire land surface. This is important in the protection of intensive, fast-changing crops. Some examples are the distribution of mites, predatory cynipides, or fungus-based preparations to limit pests, such as aphids in greenhouses; or the release of egg parasites (Trichogramma) against the corn borer.

Organic methods preserve the ecosystem. The stability of this system, vital to our survival, is especially dependent on its diversity and the complexity of its elements which all intertwine. The continual use of chemical pesticides against pests can result in a chain reaction know as "pesticide syndrome" in which the consequences are a lowering of the number of natural predators, an increase in pest damages, and the need for more and more frequent treatments. Acaricides, insecticides, and fungicides selectively effective against any single group of pests are rare. By contrast, almost all the organic agents, correctly used, spare the useful organisms.

The intense use of pesticides very often leads to the development of resistant stocks. More than 400 plant pests throughout the world are resistant to the major chemical insecticides. Also, the World Health Organization (WHO) has dropped some plans for the eradication of disease, because the disease-causing agent (malaria/mosquito) is resistant. Use of organic methods has never resulted in an acquired resistance by natural enemies.

Organic means can often—but not always—compete on a financial level with chemical means. Moreover, most long-lasting, effective introductions of useful organisms are quite inexpensive. It cost the state of California less than $5,000 to obtain and introduce the coccinella to control the lemon tree louse about 100 years ago. The value of fruit saved was close to $174 million in 1963–64. The net profit from this useful insect's activity after 100 years with no further introduction is immense. Farmers will accept mass production and the release of useful organisms only if the price is competitive with other methods. The increase in resistance to insecticides is a good stimulus, as is the immediate decrease in the population after treatment. It also is not necessary to wait days or weeks before selling the treated produce as is necessary with a chemical pesticide.

There are, however, several ostensible disadvantages to some organic methods of plant protection. In particular, *Bacillus thuringiensis*-based preparations cost more in the Third World than chemical insecticides (Franz, 1983). This price difference is much less in Europe and does not exist in the United States. The cause is not its small production cost, but price manipulation.

Also, organic agents often act more slowly than chemical pesticides, and their use frequently demands a good knowledge of both the organic agent and the pest. It is necessary, for example, to know in advance when a pest will undergo its greatest multiplication during the season in order to treat the pest with the organic agent at its youngest and most sensitive stages, or to prevent complete devastation. One must admit the organic agent may be trickier to use, take longer to react, and sometimes cost more, all of which are unattractive to the farmer who is accustomed to chemical products that are simple to use, seem to work quickly, and are inexpensive.

The shaky side of processes based uniquely on chemical means is encountered everywhere in the world. A better idea is to apply all appropriate methods—ecological, economical, and toxicological—in a sensible way, not to exterminate the harmful organisms, but to maintain them at an economically tolerable threshold (it is necessary to determine the population density at which it becomes profitable to combat the pest). In this area, organic methods have quite an important role to play.

But plant protection does not rest on organic pest control methods alone; other means support and complement them: planned succession of crops, specific care of soil, the use of cultivated plants with good resistance to diseases and pests, and, finally, an improvement in prevention, such as attracting pests to traps by way of sexual lures. Natural chemical means (for example, plant extracts), as well as artificial ones, have their place in this varied arsenal, too.

Excerpted from: *Franz, Dr. J. M. "Coccinelles contre pucerons: découvrez la lutte biologique" ("Coccinellas Against Louses: Discover the Organic Method") Les Quatre Saisons du Jardinage, no. 18, January-February 1983, pp. 60-67.*

Use of Pyrethrum

The insecticide pyrethrum, extracted from the flower of *Chrysanthemum cinerariifolium*, is effective against numerous insects that thrive in all climates but is harmless to warm-blooded animals. Treatment with pyrethrum, while clearly less powerful than treatments with other current chemical insecticides, remains much more economically advantageous. The following shows some species against which it is effective and some methods for use:

- cabbage flea-beetles: two sprayings
- cabbage white butterflies: two treatments after caterpillar hatching, taking care to wet the base of the cabbage thoroughly with the spraying
- aphids: same effectiveness as the nicotine spray, but pyrethrum treatment is more economical
- Cochylis and Eudemis: the grape bunches should be wet with the soapy spray when the caterpillar eggs are hatched

Excerpted from: *GRET (Groupe de Recherches et d'Échanges Technologiques) Fiche technique: "Techniques de production végétale"; "Lutte biologique—Le Pyrèthre insecticide" ("Methods of Vegetable Production"; "Biological Pest Control—Pyrethrum Insecticide"), Paris.*

More about Pesticides

The use of pesticides is constantly increasing in most European countries, even though authorities warn us against this trend. In certain countries, professionals can obtain useful insects, whether predators or parasites, such as the parasite for corn moth eggs (trichogram); the mite predator *Phytoseiulus persimilis*, to combat the greenhouse red spider (*Tetranychus urticae*); and the parasite wasp *Encarsia for-*

mosa for the greenhouse whitefly. These selective agents serve a smaller market than the widely popular nonecological methods.

In the long run, the market should improve for organic methods against pests, the use of plants resistant to disease and pests, and better methods of predicting insect damage. At present there is a lack of advisors at official plant protection agencies to help farmers replace systematic chemical treatments with ecologically sound methods. Therefore, the present tidal wave of highly toxic pesticides will continue as long as the cost of systematic application is cheaper than tests indicating whether the critical level of pests has been surpassed or not. Thus, the number of treatments in grain farming has increased dramatically over the past 20 years, going from one or two to seven and more in so-called progressive farming systems.

Besides all this, there are further difficulties for those who would like to commit themselves to using organic techniques. Certain representatives of the chemical industry have launched massive campaigns containing slanted, sometimes erroneous information. Some professionals even discourage organic methods by claiming that organic methods are no less expensive than other methods.

In our part of the world (Europe), less than 10 percent of the chemical products distributed are insecticides, but the problem they pose is serious. In fact, the products in this group are highly toxic and the risk of poisoning is great—for humans, for animals, for the entire environment. Anyone who worries about the impoverishment of our land will heed the call of beekeepers who note that numerous bee populations are lost throughout the year due to the secondary effects of pesticides.

Excerpted from: *Franz, Dr. J. M. "Coccinelles contre pucerons: découvrez la lutte biologique"* ("*Coccinellas Against Louses: Discover the Organic Method*") Les Quatre Saisons du Jardinage, *no. 18, January-February 1983, pp. 60-67.*

Organic Protection of Plant Life in China

In a work about the plants of southern China, the botanist Chi Hah relates how, since the beginning of the fourth century, citrus farmers in this region have bought predator-ant nests and placed them in trees to fight against parasites. The biological pest control tradition, that is, the use of living organisms to reduce pest populations, is therefore an ancient practice. It should not be surprising then that this method is used in a more modern way today to protect cultivated plants.

Western advisers from North America and Europe who came to China about 10 years ago usually recommended high-technology agrochemical methods: the intensive use of machinery, mineral fertilizers, and pesticides for better crop yields.

Fortunately, an innate wisdom coupled with a lack of funds, trained technicians, and appropriate infrastructure kept the Chinese from blindly following this advice. After an unhappy beginning with the Western ways, the Chinese now strive with increasing success to set a whole body of compatible procedures in motion, with the goals of increasing harvests and protecting plants.

Organic methods play an important role in this carefully balanced system. The requisite active and abundant labor force does not present an obstacle in China, since three-fourths of the country's population live in rural areas, and the Chinese leadership has stressed the value of manual labor. The Chinese system is particularly attuned to the use of natural organisms for pest control. Several examples (Franz, 1983) follow.

Peking duck is a famous specialty of Chinese cuisine. Few gourmet cooks, however, realize that the ducks are often raised to protect plants. Duck keepers with long poles lead large hordes of ducklings across cotton and rice fields, where the ducks destroy weeds and pests. Obviously, this is not a very selective process. All the plants that sprout near the principal crop and most of the soft insects on which the ducks feed are somehow classified as weeds or pests.

By contrast, the massive breeding and dissemination of insects and mites which directly attack pests, whether as parasites or predators, represent a much more specific process. For example, tiny egg parasites (barely one millimeter in size) of the genus *Trichogram* are produced everywhere in the country. These wasps of the Ichneumon family deposit their eggs on the eggs of pest butterflies.

Numerous communities maintain a specialized production laboratory to be able to release necessary quantities of trichograms (50,000 to 800,000 per hectare) in the fields as needed. The "production host," that is, the insect species whose eggs are used for this intensive breeding, is almost everywhere in China (a wild silkworm, usually of the genus *Antheraea* or *Philosamia*). Its caterpillars feed on a variety of foliage, and farmers and foresters can raise them in large containers without great expense.

During its pupal stage, the silkworm threads fat cocoons of a less-valued silk than the true silkworm (*Bombyx mori*). The work of the breeding stations begins with these cocoons. The workers harvest the females when they emerge from their cocoons. To obtain their eggs as quickly as possible, the worms are put through a sort of meat-chopper. The eggs, the densest part, are separated from the other tissue by running water.

At maturity, the large eggs are brought to the trichograms in the breeding laboratory so that the trichograms will lay eggs. To do this, the eggs are spread on cloth props or glued to paper. These "egg papers" are hung against the light, since parasites fly toward the light. About 60 adult trichograms can come from a single host production egg.

After several successive laboratory generations, the trichograms are brought to the field. Before they hatch, in about ten days, pieces of "egg paper" are deposited in various places (leaf piles, receptacles). The eggs must be placed in an open field so they won't be devoured by ants or other predator insects. The eggs are affixed to the plants that need protection so the small parasite wasps can go after the pest eggs when they hatch.

Trichograms have proven themselves against the corn borer, the pine moth, the sugarcane borer, the anobium (death-watch beetle), and other pests. However, one thing should be avoided: intervening with pesticides. Indeed, the trichograms—as we have learned from research at the Specialized Institute at Darmstadt—are quite sensitive to numerous fungicides and many herbicides.

These methods were recently introduced in France, Switzerland, and Germany to protect grain corn and sweet corn from the ravages of the corn borer. Since the treatment of one hectare (about 50 "egg papers") takes only half an hour, has no toxic risk, and costs much less than insecticides, it is no surprise that the farmers involved showed great interest. In spite of the climatic and crop system differences between Europe and China, there are still parallels between certain organic farming measures taken for crops. Because of this, Europe and China are making every effort to exchange their discoveries.

Attracting useful animals with special plant crops is another way the Chinese are committed to the organic protection of crops. For instance, poles covered with old leaves and isolated stalks of corn are frequently seen in the cotton fields. Pests which seek refuge on the foliage during the night are collected. Aphids appear on corn before cotton, quickly followed by their predators or parasites which are ready to migrate to the cotton if it, too, is attacked. These "corn poles," therefore, act as pest traps and predator attractants.

Microbiological methods of insect control, using diseases that strike insects, are also widely used in China. In these processes, bacteria, fungi, and viruses help to fight pests.

The development of a small factory in Shanghai which produces bacteria-based preparations (*Bacillus thuringiensis*) is the Chinese version of "high technology" agriculture. Regulated by modern production methods, bacteria develop spores in fermentation silos (receptacles where nutritive elements are brewed under controlled air and temperature conditions). The effectiveness of preparations obtained this way is due to the spores and their specific toxins which kill the pest caterpillars which absorb them.

In China, preparations of this type are as widespread as chemical insecticides in the West; certainly, these preparations act a little slower, but they have the advantage of being harmless to bees and other useful insects.

During my visit to China, the simple agricultural research in the laboratories of rural communes interested me most. The reproduction of the fungal insecticide *Beauveria bassiana* is an example.

A suitable material is treated with a culture in three stages. Only the first stage requires a slightly complicated nutritive medium of glucose, starch, and agar-agar. On a large scale, the culture is made on wheat or corn bran and other local products, first in glass receptacles then in stone jars. The fungi emit filaments (mycelia) which form reproductive organs while growing. If insects make contact with them, they are contaminated and the fungi invade their bodies.

The production of virus for fighting insects, as far as I could see, was new to China. In the Jiang Hu experimental center (Hu Bei province), I observed that this process (tested in France also, but not yet commercialized) can also be carried out under rudimentary conditions.

It is essential to have a good source of the pest in question, since all virus production requires living cells from its specific host.

One example is the Asiatic caterpillar, which lives in cotton bolls (*Heliothis armigera*). The caterpillars are fed at first on an artificial nutritive derivative which resembles chestnut pudding; then they are separated as they become active.

Next, the already fattened caterpillars are brought to contamination centers where each is put into a flask with a little nutritive medium and a drop of the virus-containing suspension. Later, the dead caterpillars are collected and soaked in water. The deposits in the preparation flasks, which are composed of encysted viruses, were used to protect more than 300 hectares of crops from damaging insects. Because of the selective action of viruses, warm-blooded animals run no risk of infection and the biological balance is not disturbed. Even the valuable silkworm caterpillars remain unharmed. Once again, crops are protected using local resources, following the laws of nature.

Excerpted from: *Franz, Dr. J. M. "La protection biologique des végétaux dans l'Empire du Milieu" ("Biological Plant Protection in China")* Les Quatre Saisons du Jardinage, *no. 18, January-February 1983, pp. 53-58.*

══════Question 2══════

Can storage losses be reduced without resorting
to pesticides?

The reduction of storage losses is becoming a top priority
in developing countries. In many regions of the developing
world, 25 to 30 percent in harvest is lost because of poor
storage conditions. Among the causes are insects, mold, and
rodents. The application of insecticides to stored grain usually
is the recommended solution to this problem. However, insecticides are only a partial solution and, in fact, present serious
disadvantages:

- When added to grain after harvest, insecticides are found in
  food in much higher quantities than when they are used on
  the crop.
- Errors in dosage are frequent and can lead to extremely high
  residual amounts.
- One of the most frequently used grain preservatives, lindane, is concentrated all along the food chain and found in
  very high concentrations in human milk.
- Insecticides cannot prevent the development of mold if grain
  is stored under poor conditions.

Moreover, it is possible to store grain properly without
insecticides. Until the nineteenth century, farmers the world
over stored their harvest without insecticides, and without
losing a large part of it. They focused on effective storing
techniques that didn't require pesticides. For example, in the
traditional grain bins of Sahel, the losses at the end of a year

are rarely greater than 5 percent (Benoit-Cattin, 1979; Grolleaud, 1980).

In the temperate countries, all farmers know that grains keep well when they are harvested and stored so that air can circulate throughout the grain pile (stored in thin layers, in gunny sacks, in ventilated silos, etc.). In tropical countries the problem is more difficult because of the humidity and high temperatures in certain seasons. But, farmers can take several simple precautions to diminish the risk of parasite attacks during storage (Stanley, 1976). They can harvest the crop only at full maturity and in dry weather. They can store the grain in its seed coat.

In Africa, millet is traditionally stored in its seed coat and is threshed as needed. The same is true for corn and rice in countries with little industrialization. Rice keeps better when still in the husk. The farmer should allow grains to dry in the sun before storing them. He can also mix sand, kaolin, or wood ashes with the grain. And he can add to grains of cowpea a small amount of peanut oil, as protection against weevils (Assion, 1979).

Traditional techniques used to fight insects, such as smoking (the grain is put on a wooden platform and a fire kindled underneath) or use of plants with the ability to repel insects, should be experimented with in a systematic manner. Additional research should bring out further uses for the storage techniques described above and show how to make them available to all (Gast and Sigaut, 1979).

When grains are stored in underground ditches, the anaerobic environment prevents insects from multiplying. The grain undergoes the beginning of fermentation which protects it from insects and mold in spite of the high humidity. In the past, grain stored in this manner kept very well for several years as long as the ditch was well protected from rain water. And, since it was considered a superior product, it often sold for a higher price than newly harvested grain (Gast and Sigaut, 1979).

Traditional methods provide good ways of storing grains and legumes while improving their nutritive value. Examples of some of these processes follow:

● Parboiling rice (the rice is soaked, partially steam-cooked, and dried) destroys all insect eggs in the grains; at the same time it causes the vitamins to concentrate deep inside the grain so that only a small part is lost during polishing (Gariboldi, 1974).

- Transforming wheat into bulgur (wheat is sprouted, partially cooked in water, dried, and coarsely ground) offers the same advantages. Furthermore, this process enriches vitamin and essential amino acid (lysine) content, and predigests starch.
- The manufacture of couscous allows wheat to be stored as semolina, protected from parasites and rodents (traditionally the couscous is kept in earthenware jars).
- The fermentation of certain legumes (soybeans in the Far East, locust bean in Africa) results in very high food values in products that can be stored for months, or even years. Soy sauce, widespread in China, Japan, and other Asian countries, is prepared by a slow fermentation process (six months to three years) and can be stored for several years. The fermentation transforms protein into readily digestible amino acids and, at the same time, destroys the trypsin inhibitor present in soybeans that makes them difficult to digest. The manufacture of the fermented sauces *soumbala* from locust bean in Africa brings similar processes into play (N'Doye, 1980).
- Fermented fish sauce (*nuoc-nam*) is a simple way to preserve fish which also prevents the loss of nutrients that is inevitable in tropical climates when fish is dried.

Supplementary Readings for Question 2

> Can storage losses be reduced without resorting to pesticides?

Effectiveness and Limitations of Traditional Grain Silos

Although traditional granaries could be improved, we must not forget that they are quite efficient in spite of a few disadvantages.

Their construction is fairly sophisticated, but these granaries have limited storage capacities and are not very flexible in their use. Should there be a bumper crop one year, it is not possible for the farmer to build extra silos rapidly. Also, because these structures are built for the storage of unthreshed grains, they do not function well in a commercial system which requires threshed grains.

As an instrument for family subsistence, the traditional silo remains a satisfactory system, especially if a few improvements are made. However, it is insufficient to meet the needs of the commercial market (Benoit-Cattin, 1979).

Excerpted from: *Benoit-Cattin, M. "Les céréales traditionnelles"* *("The Traditional Grains")* Afrique Agriculture, *no. 50, October 1979, p. 29.*

Storage of Grains in the Sahel

The secret of storing cereal grains resides both in the dryness of the grain and in the balance between temperature and humidity of the air. In the Sahel, good ventilation is generally sufficient to avoid heat risks during the long dry season and risks of mold or premature germination in the rainy season. Good ventilation is a natural result when granaries have walls made of *secco* (woven mats), when the harvest is light (as it usually is), and when the grain is stored on the stalk. It is different for *banco* granaries (pulverized and compressed earth) where the stock, especially threshed grain, is generally much larger. Here, ceiling openings or thatched roofs provide sufficient aeration.

The greatest enemies of stocked harvests are usually rodents and insects. The main deterrent against rodents is the use of a large, high platform supporting the granary on pillars. Sahelian farmers also know many natural methods to combat insects such as certain foul-smelling herbs. While these methods of storage may not be the most efficient, they do permit reliable storage conditions. In fact, polls and recent studies have shown that under current conditions, losses in supplies in traditional grain lofts in the Sahel have not exceeded 5 percent (Grolleaud, 1980).

Excerpted from: *Grolleaud, M. "Sahel: le pouvoir des greniers" ("Sahel: The Power of Silos")* Croissance des Jeunes Nations, *no. 215, March 1980, pp. 16-18.*

Preservation of Grains by Oiling

The infestation of cowpea by *Callosobruchus maculatus* first occurs in the fields and becomes more noticeable in the granaries after the harvest. Grain losses can be catastrophic for some small farmers. The larvae of the weevil *C. maculatus* penetrate the seeds as soon as they are full grown and spend the rest of their lives hollowing out galleries. Fumigation of infested stock gives good results in the fight against Callosobruchus, but it requires the mastery of a technology that small farmers do not often have.

A very simple method that is practical and lends itself to individual preference permits the farmer to protect his harvest himself without the risk of being poisoned, without the risk of residue, and with a small investment. It consists of mixing seed grain with ordinary peanut oil in the proportions of five to ten cubic centimeters of oil per kilogram of grain. Grain treated in this way can be stored for more than six months without being infested. The seeds germinate well and are free of any harmful residue (Assion, 1979).

The light oil film on the seeds produces a glue effect on the appendages (legs, wings, antennae) of mature weevils resulting in immobilization and death. A quick-drying effect on the eggs is followed by asphyxiation of the larvae due to the blocking of air passages.

Successful application of this method requires the following conditions:

• treating only those seeds which are completely dry; the presence of wet seeds in the treated stock may be harmful over time, provoking mold, fermentation, and rancidity.
• treating an average modest quantity of 20 to 40 kilograms at one time.
• storing the treated seed in a polyethylene bag, jerry can, or everyday jar, well sealed and moisture-proof.

Repeating this treatment about ten days after the first eliminates the risks of eggs escaping treatment due to their small size.

Excerpted from: *Assion, L. G. "Préservation des stocks de niébé sans résidus: l'huilage des grains" ("Preserving Cowpea Stocks without Residues: Oiling Grains") CIT—AUPELF—Université de Yaoundé (Cameroun), 10-12 May 1979, p. 1*

Storage of Grains in Silos and in Ditches in Medieval Andalucia

The objective is clear: to protect the grain against air and wind. Hence, the use of the term "matmura" (hiding place) which refers to underground pits of the Roman tradition. The digging tool is the hoe (*misha*). At the bottom of the silo a layer of straw two cubits thick (0.924 meters) is placed, and a similar layer covers the hole.

Between the wall partition and the grain, on the sides, there is more straw which has been tightly packed so that the wheat is isolated and not in contact with the silo wall partition. The silo wall is then coated to ward off parasites. Many substances are involved in making the coating: clay, wild cucumber, colocynth, lupine, dried and crushed myrtle, and olive water mixed with ashes. When this preparation is applied to the bin wall, it is said that neither rats nor weevils are able to get in.

Ingredients used for haylofts greatly outnumbered those for silo wall partitions. Such mixtures (sulfur, tar, sea squill, hellebore, white lead, henbane, and asafetida) come from an Oriental ritual where the material is powdered, wet, rewet, dried, and crushed again in order to obtain a perfect mixture. The structure of this process is as important as the ingredients in producing the desired effect (chasing rats away) since the bitter and the impermeable are important parts of it (Gast and Sigaut, 1979).

Excerpted from: *Gast, M. and Sigaut, F. "Les techniques de conservation des grains à long terme" ("Long-Term Conservation Methods for Grains") CNRS, Paris, 1979.*

Preservation of Grains in Underground Silos

We can now try to answer some of the questions about underground silos. First of all, why do people use underground silos?

It is clear that two major factors are involved: they are affordable and they can be made airtight. The latter is the more important of the two. Before the modern era, storage in an enclosed space was the only way to fight insects. Because of the great quantities of grain to be stored, underground silos were the only practical method of obtaining this protection.

Danger from insects, of course, is a function of climate, especially in humid, tropical countries where grain preservation is extremely difficult. "In Algeria," Doyere remarks, "no storage facility other than the silo is possible for storage beyond a certain length of time. The reason is not only the weevil's rapid multiplication, but also the grain's tendency to rot when kept in the open air." (Actually, these two causes are the same, since it is primarily the destructive action of the weevil that makes the grain rot. It seems that Doyere did not understand this.)

In North Africa, grain fermented in a silo is no less appreciated than ordinary grain. The fermented grain keeps well in bags and is ideal for making couscous. Furthermore, it is sold at a higher price than ordinary wheat. Similarly, the "ripening" (curing) of rice is not only accepted but desired in India.

Excerpted from: *Gast, M. and Sigaut, F. "Les techniques de conservation des grains à long terme" ("Long-Term Conservation Methods for Grains") CNRS, Paris, 1979.*

Rice Parboiling

Though statistical data are lacking, it has been estimated that more than 80 million tons of paddy (rough rice) are parboiled annually throughout the world, i.e., about one-fifth of the world's total rice crop—forecast as 403 million tons in 1982–1983.

Southeast Asia and the countries of tropical Africa have long been among the major producers of parboiled rice for consumption and export. In recent times, some countries in the Americas and in Europe have also begun producing or consuming parboiled rice. The term *parboiling* (also known as *boiling, overheating,* or *hydrothermic rice treatment*) covers the processing of the paddy before milling.

Water and heat are the two main elements in the process. After steeping followed by heating, which involves the action of steam, the rice must be dried before milling and storage. Even shelled or cargo rice may be processed in this way if special methods are used.

The purpose of the process is to produce physical, chemical, and organoleptic modifications in the cereal, with economic, nutritional, and practical advantages. The main changes caused by parboiling the paddy are:

- the water-soluble substances (vitamins and mineral salts) are dissolved and spread throughout the grain, thus altering their distribution and concentration among its various parts;
- drying will reduce the moisture content to optimal level, irrespective of the degree of moisture the paddy possessed before processing;
- the starch grains embedded in a proteinaceous matrix, constituting the endosperm mass, swell and expand until they fill up all the surrounding air spaces;

- the orderly polyhedral structure, characteristic of rice starch, is replaced by a homogeneous and compact mass of gelatinized starch;
- the protein substances are separated and sink into the compact mass of gelatinized starch, becoming difficult to distinguish under the microscope and less liable to extraction;
- the oil globules contained in the endospermic elements, formed by granular deposits of aleurone, are dissolved;
- the enzymes present in the rice kernel are partially or entirely inactivated;
- the oil-soluble substances in the germ and in the outer layer of the endosperm are to some extent dissolved and spread;
- all biological processes, whether dormant or active (germination; proliferation of fungus spores; growth of eggs, larvae, or insects; etc.), are permanently prevented.

These changes affect the results obtained during milling, storage, and subsequent cooking, and include the following:

- the milling yield is higher and the quality improved, as there are fewer broken grains;
- the grain structure becomes compact and vitreous, whether the particular variety of paddy treated possessed this texture or not, even if the texture of some caryopses was entirely or partly chalky;
- the milled rice becomes translucent and shiny;
- parboiled paddy and milled parboiled rice keep longer and better than in the raw state, as germination is no longer possible and the endosperm has a compact texture making it resistant to attacks by insects and to absorption of moisture from its environment;
- the grains remain firmer during cooking and are less likely to become sticky;
- a greater amount of water is absorbed during cooking, causing the rice to swell;
- after cooking, the rice absorbs less fat from added condiments;
- when cooked, the rice keeps longer and it will not go rancid so easily;
- the nutritional value of the rice is greater because of the higher content of vitamins and mineral salts that have spread during parboiling into the endosperm; this is even

true where polishing has removed the outer layer of the endosperm and the germ;

- after cooking, parboiled rice is more digestible because of its firm texture and consistency; the soft mass which it forms in the stomach is easily accessible to the gastric juices;
- fewer solids are left behind in the cooking water.

Excerpted from: *Gariboldi, F. "The Parboiling Process" FAO, Washington, D.C., 1974, pp. 1-2.*

Preparation of Couscous

To prepare couscous, several handfuls of semolina (called *dsis* or *cdir*) are placed on a large copper plate or *qaca* which is slanted toward the preparer at an angle of 30 to 40 degrees. Salted water is stirred in with both hands while sweeping the bottom of the plate with the fingers, as if with a rake, so that the water will be better distributed.

The right hand continues to rake the semolina while flour, then water, are sprinkled in with the left hand. The operation is repeated until the grains reach the desired thickness (2 to 3 millimeters in diameter). The couscous is then put through a sieve to remove the lumps and make the grains a uniform size.

Next it is spread out on white sheets and put in the sun to dry for six or seven days. Before it is put in jars (or in metal boxes called *gazdriya*, which are used more often), the couscous is wrapped in sheets in the sun for several days until thoroughly dry. Thus prepared, the couscous is ready. It will keep for several months or even years. It is steamed prior to consumption.

Excerpted from: *Gast, M. and Sigaut, F. "Les techniques de conservation des grains à long terme" ("Long-Term Conservation Methods for Grains") CNRS, Paris, 1979.*

Fermentation of Grains of Locust Bean

Nététou, also called *soumbala* in the Bambara language, is a black gruel made of fermented locust bean grain. It is a protein concentrate that, unfortunately, is not widely known today. However, it is a dish indigenous to North Sudanese civilization.

The Sahelian West Africans manage to satisfy a part of their protein needs with balls of *nététou* in very small quantities (N'Doye, 1980).

Another example of man's tremendous capacity for adaptation comes from Chad where the people preserve sheeps' bile from one year to the next as an ingredient in preparing pulses, to make them easier to digest.

Excerpted from: *Thianar N'Doye (Dr.) interview "La nutrition procède de la philosophie" ("Nutrition Is a Question of Philosophy")* Cérès, *no. 73, January-February 1980, pp. 17-23.*

Question 3

Do chemical products used in agriculture have a serious effect on health?

The toxic levels of chemicals used in agriculture for humans have been underestimated for a long time. Except for cases of poisoning caused by handling pesticides, it was long believed that pesticides had negligible toxic effects, and fertilizers, none at all. We now know that most adverse health conditions are due to long-term effects of exposure that show up after many years—even decades—of use. However, it is difficult to establish a cause-and-effect relationship because numerous other factors are involved.

It has now been demonstrated, however, that pesticides can have serious effects on human health (Dajoz, 1969; Aubert, 1977; Lederer, 1977). For example, the organochlorinated insecticides (DDT, HCH, lindane, heptachlorine, aldrin, dieldrin) accumulate along the food chains. In industrialized countries, very high concentrations of insecticide have been found in human milk, humans being at the end of the food chain. In France, there is an average of 5 milligrams of organochlorinated insecticide residue for each kilogram of milk-fat (some human milk contains up to 15 milligrams per kilogram compared to 0.3 milligrams per kilogram for cow's milk).

In India, human milk has, on the average, 19.5 milligrams of DDT per kilogram of fat. A breast-fed Indian baby absorbs 20 times more DDT than the daily admissible dose set by the World Health Organization (WHO) (Aubert, 1974; Pröstler, 1981). The organochlorinated insecticides, prohibited for many years in most industrialized countries, are still widely used in many developing countries.

Certain fungicides can be transformed by the body into carcinogenic substances. It has been found that the dithiocarbamates (manebe, zinebe, mancozebe) can give rise to the carcinogen, ethylene-thioure.

Handling toxic pesticides without precautions—a widespread practice in the Third World due to lack of information on the dangers of these products—can cause serious, even fatal, accidents. It is estimated that each year, throughout the world, 500,000 persons are poisoned by pesticides (Agarwal, 1978).

Fertilizers are not in themselves toxic products. Unlike pesticides which are composed primarily of molecules that do not exist in nature and that are obtained by chemical synthesis, fertilizers are either natural matter (rocks, minerals) or synthetic products composed of molecules that do exist in nature (nitrates, ammonia compounds, urea). For this reason, agronomists have long denied the toxicity of fertilizers. However, the danger of nitrates is now well established.

Nitrates transform into nitrites which can combine with numerous organic substances (natural or synthetic) to form carcinogenic nitrosamines. The carcinogenic effects of nitrates and nitrosamines are reinforced by various factors, notably: ionizing rays, synthetic estrogen, insecticides, medicine, vitamin B_1 deficiency, etc. (Armijo and Coulson, 1975). Besides their carcinogenic effects, nitrates (or products derived from them) have negative effects on the body: reproduction (birth defects and mutations), nervous system (modification of electroencephalogram, decrease in brain activity and memory), immune system reactions, glandular system (thyroid inhibition), etc.

In industrialized countries, the amount of nitrates present in food and water has risen considerably in the past 20 years, principally because of the increased use of nitrogenous fertilizer. Vegetables widely consumed in Europe, such as lettuce and radishes, contain 50 to 100 times more nitrates than the maximum allowed in drinking water (44 milligrams per liter).

The amount of nitrates in water increases regularly, with consequences that can only be measured over the long term. It can be said, therefore, that in industrialized countries nitrates carry the gravest consequences of all farming pollution. In developing countries, this problem is not yet as serious because the nitrate fertilizers are limited, but it will grow worse as the amount of nitrates increases.

Imbalanced fertilization (excessive nitrates, insufficient minerals) lowers food's nutritive value (decrease in dry weight, in amount of vitamins present, in minerals, in essential amino acids) (Scharpf and Aubert, 1976). Also, factories that produce fertilizers and especially pesticides are in themselves sources of pollution. The accident at Seveso, Italy, where unintended pollution of an area with the herbicide dioxin (an extremely toxic and teratogenic product) took place, has shown us that (Lederer, 1977; Lesca, 1980).

At first glance, the toxicity problem of chemical products used in agriculture can appear secondary to the problem of malnutrition. Experts may say that between pesticides and famine, pesticides are the lesser of two evils. However, this is a false dilemma since hunger can be overcome while greatly reducing the use of chemical products in farming (see Question 1). Even in the short term, the toxicity of pesticides is far from being negligible.

Therefore, the short-term solution to hunger that pesticides offer is nullified by their threat to the health and well-being of consumers. The resistance incited by long-term use of pesticides has also proven them a poor solution to the hunger problem.

Supplementary Readings for Question 3

> Do chemical products used in agriculture have a serious effect on health?

Toxicity of Pesticides for Man

Insecticide toxicity develops over a long period of time. Since insecticides are cumulative poisons, like heavy metals, the real danger they represent is not measurable. Insecticides have been shown to be highly toxic to a great number of animal species; they are also poisonous for man. Many statistics are available each year on the thousands of serious or fatal poisonings resulting from organophosphate insecticides.

Insecticides can be absorbed by the digestive tract when food containing these highly toxic residues is eaten. Insecticides can also be absorbed through breathing, especially when the temperature is high. Air saturated with parathion vapors, for example, contains 0.09 milligram/cubic meter at 20°C and 1.05 milligrams/cubic meter at 40°C. The maximum tolerable concentration for long exposure is only 0.1 milligram/cubic meter (Dajoz, 1969). Thus, there is considerable danger for workers who come in contact with this insecticide without a protective mask. Finally, many insecticides such as nicotine, aldrin, parathion, and HCH can even penetrate the skin. HCH is responsible for many cases of dermatosis among Argentinian workers who handle it.

One should be careful to differentiate between toxicity from one single exposure and toxicity which results from repeated contact. Quantities dangerous for man extrapolated from experiments on rabbits can be seen in table 3–1.

Table 3-1

	One application (g)	Repeated applications (g)
TEPP	0.6	0.3
Parathion	3	0.3
HCH	3	1.2
Nicotine	3	2.4
Toxaphene	46	2.4
Chlordane	113	2.4
DDT	169	9

It is evident that dangerous amounts corresponding to repeated exposures are much lower than those which correspond to a single exposure. This fact is often ignored, and too frequently only the toxicity level of an insecticide is indicated, which does not give an accurate idea of its threat. Thus, in the case of rats, DDT has an average lethal dosage of 250 milligrams/kilogram; but if the animal absorbs 0.1 milligram of DDT regularly during seven or eight months, hepatic lesions develop. Similarly, aldrin induces an inhibition of estrus and a lowering of the basal metabolic rate in the rat, with amounts as weak as those found in trace amounts in food (Ball, 1954).

Biskind (1953) has brought much data to light concerning the pathological effects of organochlorine and, in particular, DDT. According to him, a number of liver ailments and digestive and cardiovascular disorders in the United States and in certain other countries are due to the widespread use of insecticides. Biskind also found that, in general, new insecticides are used without concern for the danger they present to public health.

Furthermore, the United States Department of Health has found that DDT attacks both the spleen and the spinal cord;

biopsies on fatty tissue have shown traces of DDT in 111 of 113 persons examined. It is known that DDT is present in cow's milk in sufficient quantities to be harmful to consumers for more than three months after the cow has ingested the pesticide residue.

The increase in the death rate from exposure to organochlorine insecticides has also attracted the attention of public health specialists. Unfortunately, these health officials are often overwhelmed by manufacturers concerned with sales and by farmers concerned with increasing their harvests and profits.

Excerpted from: *Dajoz, R. "Les insecticides" ("Insecticides") Presses Universitaires de France, Collection "Que sais-je?" no. 829, Paris, 1969, p. 128.*

Scientific Proof of the Effect of Pesticides on Man and Animals

The preceding evidence, as troubling as it may be, still cannot answer the question: do the traces of pesticide that we ingest daily present a serious threat to our health? Some say yes, others no. Each side brings forth arguments which seem solid. But there has been no consensus of opinion, because experimental conclusions are lacking.

This can easily be explained: long-term cause-and-effect relationships are extremely difficult to establish. On the other hand, widespread pollution of food sources is a relatively new phenomenon in human experience: it has been observed only 30 years in the United States, and hardly more than 20 years in Europe. It is probable that very small amounts absorbed by man produce effects only after several decades of daily exposure (Aubert, 1977).

"The dosage makes the poison," said Paracelsus. In other words, a poison is only a poison after the organism has been exposed to a certain amount of it; below that, it is inoffensive, even beneficial. Even medicines contain substances which become poisonous when routine ingestion has led to a certain threshold concentration in the body. This principle, applied to pesticides, leads to the notion of "acceptable levels," below which toxicity should not occur.

This principle must be questioned, however. An experiment related to the absorption of DDT by five successive generations of mice showed no significant difference in the first two generations. However, the third generation of mice absorbing DDT exhibited a significantly higher incidence of leukemia, while cancer cases became significant with the fourth generation.

It must be stressed that mice absorb greater quantities of DDT than humans under normal conditions, but the importance of the experiment is this conclusion: certain pesticides have long-term effects that appear for the first time in the third or fourth generation of exposure.

Another example comes from the work of Druckrey and Schmahl. They administered two carcinogenic substances to groups of rats in decreasing dosages. See table 3–2 for the results with one of these substances.

Table 3-2	Relation between dosage of paradimethylaminotibene and its effect on cancer of the ear canal in rats	
Daily dosage (mg/kg)	Time necessary for appearance of tumors in 50% of animals (days)	Total dose necessary to provoke tumors in 50% of animals (mg/kg of body weight)
3.4	250	852
2.0	342	685
1.0	407	407
0.5	560	280
0.28	607	170
0.2	675	135
0.1	900	90

The figures in the third column show—contrary to the logic and principles of Paracelsus—that the amount necessary to induce cancer becomes less as the daily ingested quantity is reduced. Almost ten times less of the carcinogenic substance is needed to produce a tumor when rats absorb 0.1 milligram a day as when they absorb 3 milligrams.

Excerpted from: *Aubert, C.* L'agriculture biologique—Pourquoi et comment la pratiquer (Organic Farming—Why and How to Practice It) *Éd. Le Courrier du Livre, Paris, 1977, p. 363.*

Pesticide Poisoning—Another Third World Disease

An estimated 500,000 people throughout the world are killed or incapacitated by insecticide poisoning every year, though no detailed statistics are available. The World Health Organization (WHO) Expert Committee on the Safe Use of Pesticides, which met recently in Geneva, strongly recommended that developing countries start setting up national control agencies for registering pesticides. These agencies should not only register pesticides but also evaluate the nation's needs for new ones and control their introduction. The WHO committee also stressed the importance of health education by well-trained personnel who would go out into the field to instruct farmers in choosing pesticides, storing them, and using them safely.

For the first time, a majority of the WHO committee's members came from the Third World. Most of them agreed that little information reaches farmers and that the knowledge available is often not put to use. Most peasants and health workers continue to use replacements for DDT in the same way they used DDT. They still mix chemical solutions with their hands and carry buckets of pesticides on their heads. Changing such habits will take a long time, given the poor leadership in these countries.

The Third World can also expect some very nasty surprises with pesticides. The WHO Expert Committee on Vector Biology and Control has just reported the full details of the 1976 malathion poisoning disaster in Pakistan. Malathion is a pesticide that is considered to be relatively safe when handled properly.

More than 2,500 field workers who were spraying malathion against malaria mosquitoes were poisoned and 5 of them died. Some time elapsed before the pesticide was linked to the illness and many workers, in fear of losing their jobs, kept on working despite the risk. The incident was caused largely by failure to use elementary precautions during handling and spraying which shows, says WHO, that poor handling occurs in large-scale vector control programs in developing countries, despite clear directions and package labels. Further investigations of the pesticide samples from Pakistan revealed that their toxicity had increased considerably in recent years due to organophosphorus impurities in the malathion. These impurities inhibit enzymes in the human body which normally break down and thus detoxify malathion. This resulted in an increase of malathion's toxicity to exceptionally high levels. This contamination effect has been known for 20 years, but until the Pakistan incident the impurities were never considered of critical importance to man (Agarwal, 1978).

Excerpted from: *Agarwal, A. "Pesticide Poisoning—Another Third World Disease"* New Scientist, *London, 21-28 December 1978, p. 917.*

Pesticides and Mother's Milk in France

Another "surprise" effect of pesticides that developing countries might expect arises from the quantities of pesticides ingested by breast-fed babies of mothers who have been exposed to pesticides either directly or indirectly.

We will take the case of a three-month-old breast-fed baby, weighing 5 kilograms and drinking 900 grams of milk a day. Each day, this baby will absorb:

- 0.1 milligram of DDT or 0.02 milligram per kilogram of weight;
- 0.01 milligram of heptachloride or 0.002 milligram per kilogram of weight;
- 0.007 milligram of aldrin plus dieldrin or 0.0014 milligram per kilogram of weight;
- 0.08 milligram of HCH plus HCB or 0.016 milligram per kilogram of weight.

The comparison with the daily admissible doses approved by WHO shows that the baby will ingest:

- 4 times more DDT than the daily admissible dose (set at 0.005 milligram per kilogram);
- 4 times more heptachloride than the daily admissible dose (set at 0.0005 milligram per kilogram);
- 7 times more aldrin plus dieldrin than the daily admissible dose (set at 0.0002 milligram per kilogram).

These are only averages, however. With especially polluted milk, the quantity absorbed by the baby can be 10 times greater than the daily admissible dose. The implications of this on the health of future populations are, obviously, very serious.*

Note: The figures above are for 1971. Since then, pollution of human milk by organochlorides has appreciably diminished in France (and in all industrialized countries) because use of most insecticides of this family is prohibited. Unfortunately, the same is not true in the Third World (see chart 3).

Excerpted from: *Aubert, C. "Le lait maternel" ("Human Milk") Nature et Progrès, October-November-December 1974, pp. 21-29.*

Mysterious Diseases

High over the Deccan plateau in India, some 350 kilometers away from Bangalore city (the capital of the southern state of Karnatka), sits the small town of Sagar. Off the main east-west state highway, you dip deep into the slope of a valley, encircled on all sides by dense forests. In the open, there is a panorama as picturesque as southern California's—studded with verdant fields, canyons, and wild foliage of wonderful hues.

The Green Revolution came to this area a decade ago. Once a very backward part of the country, it was transformed almost overnight by technology. Modern ways took hold of the progressive farmers. Tractors replaced ox-drawn plows, mechanization began to revitalize agriculture. New lands were cleared for cultivation, a high-yielding strain of rice was introduced, and new crops—areca nut, pepper, cardamom, and coffee—were planted. Pests, naturally, swarmed in, so chemicals were pumped in just as quickly to combat them. A

Chart 3
Pollution of Human Milk by DDT in Different Countries

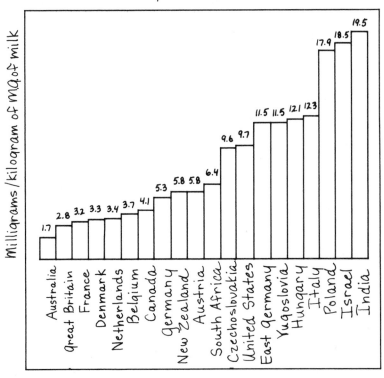

Excerpted from: Pröstler, E. "Stillen trotz verseuchter Umwelt", Öko-Institut, Dreisam-Verlag Freiburg, 1981.

wide variety of pesticides—endrin, parathion (folidol), malathion, quinolphos, carbofuran, and so on—were sprayed. Endrin and folidol, which have long-lasting residual effects on crops, were copiously administered.

The residue was as instantaneous as it was devastating. The fields, being in the heavy rainfall area—around 250 to 300 centimeters a year—retained the chemical toxicity. The rice paddies and the pond water were contaminated. Mass death of fauna—fish, crabs, and frogs—followed.

The ecological balance of the human habitat was also disturbed. The defoliation of the trees surrounding the fields removed the subsoil's moisture-retaining cover. The natural nutrients of the good earth dwindled as soil erosion occurred. Indeed, the topography of the land itself changed. The whole environment—air, water, even food—was polluted.

"Prosperity," however, continued as production and productivity mounted. Paddies were producing 1.4 to 1.9 tons of rice per hectare as opposed to 0.5 to 0.7 previously. In the upland irrigated areas, the yield increased to as much as 10 tons, averaging 5 tons per hectare (Roy, 1978).

Eventually, the environment retaliated with a vengeance. The economic needs of the new agriculture had already altered human relationships. High costs of equipment, seeds, fertilizers, and chemicals could no longer support the old farm workers. Landless people became jobless when the soil gave out. The farm worker used to receive food as part of his wages; now all he knew was hunger. Never robust, he weakened further and desperation drove him to catching and eating crabs, the same crabs filled with the concentrated chemicals spread earlier in the flooded rice paddies. Soon, a mysterious disease afflicted his body.

The disease was unknown and, therefore, was named *Handigodu* Syndrome after the village where it first occurred. It was a disease of the joints that was first observed about six years ago, with its maximum incidence occurring two years later.

Handigodu Syndrome was, for the most part, confined to a few villages around the towns of Sagar in Shimoga district and Balehonnur in Chikmagalur district. It was seen predominantly among the Hrijans, who are mostly dispossessed, poor agricultural workers. Out of a total population of 130,000 in the Sagar area, the Hrijans numbered about 12,000. A study revealed that at its peak in 1975–1976, the disease attacked more than 34 villages with no less than 300 patients. Given the type of medical facilities available in India, it is entirely possible that not all the cases were reported to the authorities, nor were all the patients hospitalized. However, 36,700 people were examined in the stricken areas and a door-to-door check was carried out to detect cases. The disease seems now to have subsided, since no new cases have been reported in the past year or so.

The onset of the disease is gradual, beginning with mild pain in the lower limbs, particularly in the lumbosacral regions, hips, and knee joints. The pain later increases, sometimes leading to immobility. A few people suffered from crippling deformities of the joints. In 40 of the 60 affected households that were investigated, more than one member of the family was a victim. Men, women, and children between the ages of 6 and 50 were affected, with the children often becoming ill first. The villages in the valley still bear the burden of these living corpses, the victims of a despoiled environment; the skeletal heads, the sunken faces with motionless eyes, the rickety torsos—all are the result of senseless practices.

Epidemiological studies suggest that the disease was precipitated by certain changes in the microecological system. The hazards of the deadly pesticides' residues entering the human food chain are obvious enough. The only positive side of this story seems to be the promising research being done at the National Institute of Nutrition, Hyderabad, to determine the disease's cause, as well as its prevention and cure.

Excerpted from: *Roy, P. "Des maladies mystérieuses" ("Mystery Disease—No Mystery")* Mazingira, the International Journal of Environment and Development, *Tyrooly International Publishing Ltd., Dublin, Ireland, no. 6, 1978, pp. 74-77.*

Nitrates and Cancer

Another disease—cancer—can also be traced to farming methods in Chile, which has the world's second highest death rate from stomach cancer (Armijo and Coulson, 1975). The death rate in 25 provinces over a 15-year period has been analyzed, and a geographic location where the death rate is greatest from stomach cancer has been determined.

Three agricultural provinces (Maule, Linares, and Nuble) which use a great deal of nitrate fertilizers have a population of 460,000 and average death rates of 50.1 per 1,000,000. At the other end of the country, approximately 3,000 miles away, the death rate is half that of the above provinces.

Thirty percent of all cancer deaths are attributed to stomach cancer. In order to link these effects to precise causes in the Chilean provinces, correlations were made with socioeconomic variables. There was a strong correlation between the death rate and exposure to nitrate fertilizers.

It seems that there was no link between the concentration of nitrates in water deemed "drinkable" and the death rate from stomach cancer. On the other hand, a clear correlation seemed to exist between amounts of nitrate fertilizer applied in the area and this same mortality. It is probable that food was the source of the contamination, since crops can accumulate a high nitrate concentration when excess nitrogen fertilizer is made available to the plants. Once they have entered the stomach, these nitrates can then be converted to carcinogenic nitrosamines.

Excerpted from: *Armijo, R. and Coulson, A. "Épidémiologie du cancer de l'estomac au Chili: le rôle des engrais azotés" ("Epidemiology of Stomach Cancer in Chile: The Role of Nitrogen Fertilizers")* International Journal of Epidemiology, *vol. 4, no. 4, 1975, p. 1.*

Dioxin in Herbicides

A final example of the effect that pesticides have had on human health comes from Vietnam where the American army spread two defoliants, 2,4-D (dichloramine) and 2,4,5-T, in an attempt to starve the Vietcong population. A warning cry was sounded when birth defects were found in newborn children as well as animals in the area. Defects occurred during experiments that were carried out. But what was striking about these defects was their inconsistency; it seemed that an impurity had to be the cause.

Wade (see Lederer, 1977) isolated an impurity in 2,4,5-T that he felt was responsible for the defects. It was 2,3,7,8 tetra-chloro-dibenzo-para dioxine. He further established that it was responsible for the teratogenous action observed in all the chlorophenol herbicides.

This product caused the danger in the case of the accident at Seveso (see Question 3). Massive formation of 2,3,7,8-T instead of 2,4,5-T occurred when industrial equipment used for synthesis was heated too high. A leak then spread it throughout the area. The defoliant 2,3,7,8-T is not only highly toxic but is also very persistent. At present, there is no effective means of assuring its destruction, and its effects on future generations remain unknown.

Excerpted from: *Lederer, J.* Alimentation et Cancer (Food and Cancer) *Éd. Nauwelaerts/Maloine, Louvain/Paris, 1977.*

Question 4

To what degree does the development of export crops endanger the health of Third World populations?

Export crops have totally upset traditional agrarian systems (Dupin and Brun). Before the introduction of cash crops destined for exportation, all cultivated land and all time devoted to agriculture were used for food production. Now, however, the land area used for food production is shrinking or at least not growing at the same rate as the population. In Brazil, for example, the land allotted to beans, a popular staple with rice and a source of essential protein, decreased by 36 percent in five years (from 1967 to 1972) in favor of cash crops, principally cotton and soybeans. The best places in crop rotations are often reserved for cash crops; and in areas with continuous cultivation, the soil has less time to rest and, therefore, is gradually exhausted. Fertilizers and pesticides are used mainly on export crops.

For all these reasons, food crop yields have stood still or declined, while export crop yields have greatly increased almost everywhere during the last 20 years. In Mali, between 1960 and 1972, sorghum production decreased from 1,000 to 800 kilograms per hectare while cotton production went from 480 to 800 kilograms per hectare. In addition, the land allotted to cotton increased from 26,000 to 90,000 hectares. It can be said, therefore, that exports are directly responsible for malnutrition both by exhausting and polluting the soil and by displacing land formerly used for growing food crops. All

69

these factors contribute to the increasingly poor health of the population.

Export crops have also upset social structures and economic relations. Unequal distribution of revenue created by export crops and lowered availability of subsistence crops have caused an increase in staple food prices so the poor can no longer afford to buy them. Export crops have also largely contributed to the indebtedness of poor people who must buy seeds, fertilizers, and products necessary for their crops on credit. Solidarity and village interdependence have given way to the pursuit of profit and "every man for himself." In general, export crops are tended by men. Because the men neglect the growing of food crops in deference to their cash crops, the women's work load has increased, cutting into the time they have to spend on their other duties as wives and mothers (Malick, 1976).

Solving these socioeconomic problems, however, does not lie in eliminating export crops. The elimination of export crops is neither possible nor desirable, but we must begin to integrate them into a balanced production system, paying equal attention to food crops (Provent and Ravignan, 1977).

Supplementary Readings for Question 4

> To what degree does the development of export crops endanger the health of Third World populations?

Development of Export Crops to the Detriment of Food Crops

The interaction of cash crops and food crops is complex, and it cannot be denied that the first has had favorable effects on the second in certain circumstances. However, to a larger extent, the emphasis placed on cash crops—peanuts, cotton, coffee, cocoa, pineapple, tea, hemp, etc.—has been disastrous for food crops like rice, millet, yams, and cassava. The percentage of land used in raising food crops, cash crops for the local market, and export crops varies according to geographical location. According to a U.N. report in the early 1960s, export crops occupied 45 percent of cultivated land in Ghana and only 2 percent of cultivated land in Kenya.

Many examples can be cited of the replacement of food crops by cash crops. In the Central African Republic, sorghum was replaced by cassava, which was easier to grow, but had less nutritive value. French colonial policies then introduced rubber, followed by cotton, both of which lowered food production to an alarming level. To obtain higher yields, cotton was cultivated on reclaimed land and given priority in crop rotations.

While cotton was sown at the same time as food crops such as millet, because cotton cultivation took much more work, the food crops tended to be neglected.

In many countries, the effort to popularize cash crops arises from the government's desire for increased tax revenues. The peasant farmer complains that he no longer has time to plant millet, while both producer and wage-earner are becoming more and more dependent on world markets. For example, in the south of Ghana from 1900 to 1920, cocoa replaced cassava, yams, and plantains. The new cocoa harvest was worth so much more that the peasant found he could buy more provisions than he could produce for himself.

Similarly, the standard of living for the peanut farmer is directly linked to the price of this commodity in the world market as well as to the price of imported products such as cereals (especially rice), other foodstuffs, and manufactured products which the farmer must now purchase.

The current drop in exchange rates, therefore, not only affects the budgets of entire countries which are dependent on a single crop, but also determines the standard of living, hence the standard diet, of small producers, individuals, or employees.

Excerpted from: *Dupin, H. and Brun, T.* "Évolution de l'alimentation dans les pays en voie de développement" ("Evolution of Food in Developing Countries") Développement et Santé, no. 11, p. 11.

Disadvantages of Export Crops

Experts have reported as early as the 1950s that there are disadvantages to intensive farming for export (Wenger, 1974). For example, the intensive peanut planting of Senegal or the cotton planting in tropical Africa have shown the disturbances that can be created by the introduction of commercial farming into a traditional system. Using erosion as one example, we will quote a passage of *We Have Only One Earth* by Barbara Ward and Rene Dubois:

> *It is estimated that 92.8 tons per hectare of soil
> have been destroyed in one area of the Ivory Coast
> where woods were cleared for cassava cultivation; in
> an adjacent forest in 1956, the earth lost only 2.1 tons
> of soil per hectare. Likewise, in one part of Senegal
> where woods were cleared for peanut cultivation,
> erosion took place at 14.9 tons per hectare while only
> 0.02 ton per hectare was eroded in a neighboring
> forest.*

Commercial crops (cotton, for example) were cultivated to
the detriment of food crops since they were not associated or
intercropped with the latter. This greatly diminished soil
fertility before anyone had ascertained that there would be
sufficient yields for local food consumption.

Trends such as this have lead experts to question the
intensity and negligence of the systems under which cash
crops are now grown. "With these policies," says Professor
Lemee, "world cotton production has reached great heights,
but for how long? And with how heavy a mortgage has the
future of the country been burdened?"

Excerpted from: *Wenger, E. "Environnement et Tiers-Monde
africain" ("Environment and the African Third World")* Le Mois
en Afrique, *no. 102, Paris, 1974, pp. 36-37.*

Senegal and the Peanut

An example of the intensive cash-cropping that can displace local food crops is the cultivation of peanuts in Senegal.

In 1638 France established its first settlement at Saint
Louis, Senegal. At that time, the peanut, which came from
Mexico and Brazil, was unknown in Senegal; it arrived some
years later, introduced by slave traders. The first peanut
exports, totaling 722 kilograms, took place in 1840. Three
years later, exports were up to 185 tons. But after 1885 with
the construction of the first railroad, production was organized on a larger scale, around the railroads and ports—Dakar,
Rufisque, Kaolak—and then around the Sine-Saloum region,
making up the "peanut-triangle" or "useful Senegal"
(Legarrec, 1979).

In the beginning, peasants were pressured by the colonial

army to cultivate a crop that was not traditional; the growth of the peanut market proceeded "naturally," that is, practically without force. In 1860, this movement was boosted by a tax payable in cash, on the advice of General Gallieni. As the peanut was their only salable commodity, the peasants were obliged to grow it to obtain the necessary money to pay their taxes or debts to revenue agents.

Sally N'Donogo, of the General Union of Senegalese Workers in France, has lived in a Puteaux housing project since 1956. He is the author of several books that evoke the old days and colonization in Senegal. "Before the peanut, each village was self-sufficient and to a certain extent self-ruling. The inhabitants cultivated millet, sorghum, corn, sweet potatoes, and whatever cotton they needed for themselves. They relied on stored millet during slack seasons. There were also small local manufacturers: women spun cotton, men wove, blacksmiths made tools necessary for the community in their own foundries. The land was not drained of minerals because crops were rotated and fertilizer was not needed. The peanut began with forced labor; but colonizers soon created new 'needs' in the local markets, such as new fabrics. 'Luxury' began to invade the country. At the tax exchange office, it was so many kilograms of peanuts traded for so many meters of cloth or so much money—half barter, half money. Socioeconomic systems that existed before began to be done away with in favor of the peanut crop. The peasants did not keep the money they were given. They soon spent it paying taxes or debts, for they had no cushion between the two harvests: there were no longer any millet lofts, for millet had disappeared in favor of the peanut. Farmers went into debt, and those who could no longer get by, left for the slums of Dakar, then for France."

At the time of independence in 1960, the Senegalese inherited the colonial system, which consisted of 50 percent of the land being used for peanuts, which extended more and more toward the most drained land. There is such a lack of food crops in Senegal today that one-fourth of what is needed for subsistence is imported and rice tends to replace millet, the traditional crop. Confronted with the political choice of satisfying the needs of its citizens or occupying a place in the world peanut market, the Senegalese government, while announcing plans to develop food crops, has chosen to compete in the world peanut market.

Excerpted from: *Legarrec, E. "La grande bataille des oléagineux"* ("The Great Battle of Oil Seeds") Le Monde Diplomatique, no. 299, February 1979, pp. 16-17.

Decline of Domestic Food Crops in Mexico

A decline in the production of domestic food crops has also been seen in Mexico where the amount of land planted in soybeans, safflower, and livestock feed has increased dramatically. Table 4–1 shows the unevenness of Mexican agriculture resulting from the agro-industrialization of certain areas, where 82.7 percent and 74.9 percent of the best irrigated land is reserved for "star" crops, including soybeans and safflower.

Basic food crops become less and less available as they are replaced by crops intended for the agricultural market (see table 4–2). However, raising beef, pork, and poultry continues to progress. In 12 years, the amount of livestock as well as the number of pigs raised has almost doubled in Mexico (Lopez, 1978). In order to nourish livestock, mash and other feeds are made from soybean, safflower, alfalfa, and sorghum. As investments in livestock surpass those made in agriculture, the meat and meat by-products industries as well as the dairy industry are undergoing considerable expansion, at the expense of basic food crops. Needless to say, small farmers in Mexico are rarely able to afford the products derived from their country's fast-growing meat-packing and dairy industries.

Mexico, therefore, the cradle of the Green Revolution, has become an importer of grains and agricultural raw materials. Agricultural research has improved seeding techniques greatly. But growth in productivity requires more than improved seeding: it requires fertilizers, insecticides, pesticides, tractors, and machines. These technological components of the Green Revolution must be imported and thus, a new form of dependency has been created. This is ironic for a country that the Green Revolution was supposed to have liberated from the need to import grains.

The "multinationalization" of agriculture means that Ford Motor Company, International Harvester Company, Massey

Table 4-1   Priority for development of "star" crops

	1960	1965	1970	1975
Corn	100.0	164.7	163.6	143.3
Wheat	100.0	181.2	225.5	234.7
Black beans	100.0	162.5	174.8	169.2
Rice	100.0	115.3	134.8	168.8
Safflower	100.0	248.5	899.6	857.5
Soybean	100.0	164.0	4,309.6	11,536.7
Sorghum	100.0	356.9	1,313.7	1,503.9
Alfalfa	100.0	134.9	217.8	280.5

Source: Secretaria de agricultura, dirreccion general de Economia Agricola, COCOSA.

Table 4-2   Decline of food available per inhabitant

	1960	1970	1975
Basic products* (millions of tons)	11.4	11.8	12.9
Population (millions of inhabitants)	34.9	48.3	60.2
Availability per inhabitant (kilograms)	0.326	0.244	0.214

*Corn, black beans, and wheat.

Ferguson Inc., and John Deere together produced and exported 70,000 tractors to Mexico between 1966 and 1977. Seeds for sorghum, soybean, and safflower cultivation as well as fertilizers were furnished by Northrup King Company, DeKalb, Asgrow Seed Company, and Dow Chemical Company. From

1960 to 1977, Anderson, Clayton & Co. and Ralston Purina Co. manufactured feed for livestock, while Cargill, Inc., Bunge Corp., Cook International, Inc., and Mitsubishi International Corp. furnished 17.8 million tons of basic agricultural products. Nestle's production of milk and dairy products grew from 23,800 tons in 1960 to 70,483 tons in 1974. From the above statistics, it is easy to see who the true beneficiaries of "multinationalization" of agriculture are.

The resulting industrialization of agriculture has also had ecological consequences. The northeast irrigation zone (Tamaulipas), which is the principal sorghum-production region in Mexico, has an irrigation capacity of 280,000 hectares. At present, 80,000 hectares have become sterile due to salinization and 64,000 additional hectares are about to undergo the same fate. The situation is identical in the irrigated zones in the northwest (Sinaloa, Sonora, and Baja, California), principal producers of soybeans and safflower; 172,000 hectares became useless for farming due to poor utilization of water and poor draining methods.

As a whole, the intensive agriculture practiced in the irrigated zones in the northeast, northwest, and center of the country has caused the loss of 600,000 hectares, made unproductive after salinization. More than 700,000 hectares will soon have to be abandoned for the same reason.

By 1974, the World Bank had lent up to $195.5 million to restore some of the land which was lost (Lopez, 1978). Soon, however, this same land will be used for the same practices of "multinational" agriculture, thereby continuing the vicious circle of destruction.

Excerpted from: *Musalem Lopez, O. "Mexique: une forme de multinationalisation" ("Mexico: A Form of Multinationalization")* Le Monde Diplomatique, *no. 294, September 1978, pp. 14-16.*

Social Consequences
of Export Crop Development

The cohesiveness of family work is becoming more difficult to maintain, for young adults refuse to be confined to food-crop farming which is not remunerative. They also refuse to be employed on land owned by their elders and thus to be confused with foreign labor. The solution is to leave for the city unless the elder gives them a piece of land on which they will be able to do remunerative farming. In other words, more and more land is being tilled for export crops, at the expense of food crops.

Excerpted from: *Comité d'Information Sahel "Qui se nourrit de la famine en Afrique?" ("Who Is Feeding on the Famine in Africa?")* Petite Collection Maspéro, no. 153, Paris, 1975, p. 200.

Increase in the Women's Workload

A semimodern agriculture, exclusively geared toward the domestic or international market, is gradually replacing traditional agriculture (based primarily on grains) that only aimed to satisfy family needs.

Subsistence crops which are less profitable are neglected or left solely to the care of women and children, while men devote themselves to profitable crops. When climatic and ecological conditions are not favorable to cash crops, the male population migrates, looking for better land, abandoning the women and children to the village. The consequences? An increase in women's work.

Before the intensive introduction of cash crops, men participated in growing grains. Once the granaries were filled enough to provide the needs of a farming year (the period between two harvests) and the taxes were paid, men had fulfilled their contract to their family and society.

The women, on the other hand, had to grind the family ration of millet every day and prepare the meal usually eaten together with the entire family. They were also responsible for finding water and wood for heat, and for the condiments and vegetables necessary to their diet. In the evening, they had to card and spin the cotton harvested on their plot of land or bought at the market in order to dress the entire family.

The introduction of cash crops has, consequently, given additional work to women (Malick, 1976). Their duties in subsistence production have now increased and they often work with their children and husbands in the cultivation of cash crops, as well as feed and clothe the family and maintain the house and surrounding yard and garden area.

Excerpted from: *Malick, S. "Un projet d'allègement du travail des femmes au Mali" ("A Project to Lighten Women's Workload in Mali") Les carnets de l'Enfance, no. 36, "Alléger le travail des femmes," UNICEF, Geneva, October-December 1976, pp. 66-86.*

Changes in Rural Zones in Tanzania

The basic difference between Tanzania's rural life now and in the past stems from the widespread introduction of cash-crop farming. Over large areas of the country, peasants spend at least part of their time—and sometimes the larger part of it—on the cultivation of crops for sale; crops like cotton, coffee, sisal, pyrethrum, and so on. But in the process, the old traditions of living together, working together, and sharing the proceeds have often been abandoned. Farmers tend to work as individuals, in competition and not in cooperation with their neighbors. And in many places the most intelligent and hard-working peasants have invested their money (or money advanced through public credit facilities) in clearing more land, extending their acreage, using better tools, and so on, until they have quite important farms of 10, 20, or even more acres. To do this, they have employed other people to work for them. Sometimes—but, unfortunately, not always—they have paid the government minimum wages to these laborers for the period over which they were employed. The result has been an increase in production for the nation as a whole—that is, an increase in the amount of wealth produced in Tanzania—and a still further increase in the wealth of the man who owned, managed, and initiated the larger farm.

The work of such people as this has shown that in the rural areas of Tanzania it is possible to produce enough crops to give an agricultural worker a decent life, with money for a good house and furniture, proper food, some reserve for old age, and so on. But the moment such a man extends his farm to the point where it is necessary for him to employ laborers in order to plant or harvest the full acreage, then the traditional system of ujamaa has been killed. For he is not sharing with other people according to the work they do, but simply paying them in accordance with a laid-down minimum wage. The final output of the farm on which both employer and employees have worked is not being shared. The money obtained from all the crops goes to the owner; from that money he pays "his" workers. And the result is that the spirit of equality between all people working on the farm has gone—for the employees are the servants of the man who employs them. Thus, we have the beginnings of a class system in the rural areas. Also, the employees may well be paid for working during harvest or during weeding but get no money for the rest of the year.

Excerpted from: *Nyerere, J. K.* Freedom and Socialism. *Oxford University Press, Oxford, 1968, pp. 342-43.*

═══ Question 5 ═══

> Is it desirable to depend on large-scale, mechanized production to solve a country's food problems?

In twentieth century industrialized countries, food production increases have paralleled mechanization and increases in the size of farm operations. But the cause-and-effect relationship is not as clear as it first appears. Mechanization and concentration have increased production per worker at a greater rate than production per surface unit. Fertilizers and the best seed varieties have been primarily responsible for land area production increases.

Nevertheless, highly industrialized, highly intensive farming operations are often cited as examples to follow, certainly in industrialized countries. However, these models are not easy or practical to copy in other parts of the world.

In Western Europe, these large, industrialized farms have a higher productivity due to the use of the best seed varieties, fertilizers, and pesticides as well as to the expert technical level of the managers. But even in highly industrialized countries, such farms are economically more vulnerable than small family farms.

In developing countries, which rarely have a sufficient industrial infrastructure, large mechanized farms are often doomed to failure. The production per hectare is almost always better in small units since crops grown on small farms are often given better care. For example, in Colombia the production per hectare is 14 times higher on small farms than on large ones. In Argentina, it is 8 times greater (Strahm, 1977).

Large mechanized farms in developing countries may present several serious economic and social problems (Mazoyer, 1982). A few of these follow:

- They encourage depopulating the rural areas in favor of overpopulated cities where unemployment is high.
- They consume more energy and more industrial products (mostly imported) than small farms, although their output may be the same.
- They increase the risk of pollution, since for the most part they produce only one crop and use many more pesticides than small farms.
- They are dependent on economic variables: price fluctuations in farm products; price increases for oil, fertilizers, and machines.
- They are more at the mercy of the weather than small farms. In case of a bad harvest, the small farmer will reduce his spending while the large farmer, whose fixed prices are much higher, risks being driven into bankruptcy.
- They aggravate social inequalities and create an underpaid rural proletariat.

Small farms are also much better adapted to low-cost methods that help to increase yields. These methods (intercropping, varied rotation, recycling of organic matter, etc.) can be tailored to each individual case. They allow the farmer to use naturally available resources to achieve sustainable crop yields and to maintain or improve soil quality.

The development of mechanical systems to facilitate man's labor is beneficial. But going from the hoe to the tractor without a transition period is an absurdity. Even industrial countries are beginning to recognize the disadvantages of rushing the mechanization process. They realize that for certain work, animals are less costly and better adapted to the job (for example, for work demanding little power on small farms). This will become more and more evident with the inescapable increase in motor fuel costs.

Supplementary Readings for Question 5

> Is it desirable to depend on large-scale, mechanized production to solve a country's food problems?

The Disadvantages of Mechanization

The problem of mechanization is crucial, because African elites are seduced by the idea of modern machines. It is difficult to convince them that agricultural progress does not depend on immediate and complete mechanization. In Guinea, the Soviet experts have used this tendency to their advantage. "How can peasants make any progress with the *daba*? Why should we not relieve them of this hardship?" It is not that mechanization is impossible on African soil. Machines will be in wide use in the future. But there are still too many obstacles. Later, I will discuss ways to get around them.

Forests cleared for cultivation by peasants have roots left in the soil and large unburned tree trunks on the ground. "They look more like a battlefield than a Belgian field," a Belgian agronomist in the Congo told me. The savanna also has numerous bushes and shrubs. The fragile topsoil is quickly destroyed by machines, as has been the case in the tobacco plantations in the northern Republic of the Congo (Brazzaville). The price of buying modern equipment and transporting it into the bush is high. If the whole African countryside was mechanized at once, the governments would be completely without foreign exchange to equip factories. Yet factories, safe under their roofs, operate year-round, while tractors, particularly in the tropics, can often work only a few weeks out of the year. Highly qualified mechanics are needed to maintain them. These are still largely Europeans, and therefore expensive. Above all, tractors increase rural unemployment.

Use of tractors has been uneconomical everywhere: in Boulel-Kaffrine, the center of mechanized peanut cultivation in Senegal, where they still scrape off the topsoil when they fell trees; at Loudima in the Congo; on the rice plantations in the Niger valley (Guinea, Mali, Niger) and the Logone valley (Chad, the Cameroons); and at the CRAM in Madagascar. From 1945–1950 the tractor was thought capable of solving all the agricultural problems of the Africans. In actual fact, it allows you to produce a peanut crop at a much higher cost in local currency than with the *daba* and manpower alone. The amount of foreign exchange necessary to mechanize an independent country, with an independent monetary system and a subsistence economy, which exports very little (Guinea), would be much more disastrous.

Current economic policy in Africa is unhealthy because it relies on foreign aid: "This money didn't cost us anything, who cares if it doesn't bring in much." Development demands that it bring in a great deal. A whole series of agricultural and general advances must be made before mechanization can logically be introduced. On the other hand, draft animals, wherever feasible, present only advantages, and can achieve the intermediate stage in agriculture, often the most useful and indispensable.

Excerpted from: *Dumont, R.* False Start in Africa, *André Deutsch, London, 1968, pp. 58-59.*

Ecosystems: Victim of Mechanization

Another factor that should be kept in mind is that the ecosystem of cleared forest and savanna is easily victimized by mechanization. These cleared lands have left a fragile soil structure behind which is easily damaged by the large machines that have sprung up to clear the land and farm the new terrain "profitably."

These operations of clearing the land rarely lead to rational and productive land development, since little thought is given to the groups living here or to soil conservation on these "unlimited," "virgin" spaces. Most often, these are "mining" farming operations whose short-term profits hide the destructive long-term effects (Mazoyer, 1982).

Victims of these operations are most often the ecosystems: the forest and savanna ecosystems of hunters and gatherers (Amazon), the prairies and the steppes of nomad and seminomad herders (Middle East, Sahel, Central Asia), the forests worked by farmers who clear the land by burning (intertropical Africa). They are victims of people who are unaware of the soil's fragile qualities.

Excerpted from: *Mazoyer, M. L. "Impasses et perspectives" ("Impasses and Perspectives") in "Le Point Critique" dir. by Morazé, C., "Sciences et techniques au service du développement agricole," l'IEDES: Collection Tiers-Monde, PUF, 1982. Cited with the author's permission.*

American Agriculture and Energy Use

The American agricultural system is a huge consumer of energy: the production of one food calorie requires ten calories of energy, if you count as well the energy that goes into production supplies and food distribution. If all countries adopted this system, 80 percent of the total energy currently consumed in the world would be just enough for the production and commercialization of food products.

Still, this percentage underestimates the energy cost of the American food production system, the watchword of which is the replacement of farm work with industrial processes (fertilizer production, tractor manufacture). While 15 percent of nonagricultural workers are employed in the food industry, a growing proportion of the costs of urbanization, including those of transportation to work, can be attributed to industrialized, agriculture-related work (Perelman, 1978).

It is also necessary to consider the enormous costs of the effects on the environment. Each year, more than one billion pounds of pesticide are spread on the soil of the United States. For each pound of food served on American tables, an average of 30 pounds of farmland is lost to erosion.

In spite of its incomparably rich land, the United States does not rank first in crop yields per hectare. For example, Switzerland and Austria have double yields for wheat; Greece

surpasses the United States in rice; Austria produces 20 percent more corn per hectare. And American crop yields would
be even lower if the best soils in the country were not cultivated.

We have seen, furthermore, that the yield of large, expensive farming operations falls below the American average. The
phenomenon is strikingly illustrated by the relationship between the net revenue and the area of land that is farmed (see
table 5–1): if all operations reached the same yields, the
figures of columns 1 and 5 would be proportional. In fact, the
small farms have a higher revenue per acre.

Table 5-1   The largest operations do not give the best
yields (total percentage for U.S.)

1 Cultivated surface in acres	2 Gross receipts	3 Production expenses	4 Pesticide expenses	5 Net revenue
6	2.7	3.7	2	7
5	3	3.2	2	4.6
7	5.9	5.6	5	7.9
14	11	10.1	11	14.5
22	20	18.4	22	24.6
46	57.3	59	57	41.4

Source: U.S.D.A. Economic Research Service.

Excerpted from: *Perelman, M. "Le modèle est-il si efficace?" ("Is
the Model So Effective?")* Le Monde Diplomatique, *no. 294, September 1978, pp. 6-7.*

The Small Farmer Is
the Most Productive

In developing countries, the fact that the small farmer is
generally more productive than the large farmer is particularly striking. A study of Argentina, Brazil, Colombia, Ecuador, and Guatemala found small farmers to be 3 to 14 times

more productive per acre than the large farmers. In Thailand, plots of 0.8 to 1.6 hectares yield almost 60 percent more rice per hectare than farms of 56 hectares or more (Moore Lappé and Collins, 1977).

There is no need to romanticize small producers. They get more out of the land precisely because they are desperate to survive on the meager resources allowed them. Small farmers plant more closely than would a machine. They mix and rotate complementary crops and they choose a labor-intensive combination of crops and livestock. Above all, they work their limited resources to the fullest. The large holders, for whom land is not the basis of daily sustenance, invariably underutilize their land.

Excerpted from: *Moore Lappé, F. and Collins, J. "Les huit mythes de la faim" ("The Eight Myths of Hunger")* Cérès, no. 58, July-August 1977, pp. 24-30.

Production of Small and Large Farms in Colombia and Argentina

One of the reasons for the poor food crop production in the Third World is the inefficient development of large landholdings. In Colombia, 66.1 percent of arable land belongs to 3.6 percent of landowners; in Argentina, 74.9 percent to 1.78 percent of landowners. These large landholdings are clearly not put to use as well as the small ones.

In Colombia, the yield per hectare is 14 times greater on the small farms than on the larger ones; in Argentina, small operations have revenues that are 8 times greater than that of large farms (Strahm, 1977).

Large portions of huge estates are not cleared for farming. Their owners are not interested in intensive farming and refuse to invest in agriculture; often they reside in town and invest their farming profits in real estate or industry located in the city, or in luxury consumer goods.

In Asia small landholdings have better crop yields as well, for the work there is more intense and the incentive to produce is greater. This same phenomenon can also be observed in the Soviet Union.

Excerpted from: *Strahm, R. H. "Pourquoi sont-ils si pauvres?" ("Why Are They So Poor?")* A la Baconnière/La Déclaration de Berne, *Neuchâtel, 1977, p. 147.*

==== Question 6 ====

Are there ways to develop irrigation programs
that are not harmful to the general health?

Agricultural progress depends upon water control in
many countries. Therefore, irrigation justly holds an important place in development programs. Large dams have permit-
ted the irrigation of a great amount of soil, but they have had
unforeseen consequences. Because the presence of water favors the development of numerous parasitic diseases (malaria,
onchocercosis, schistosomiasis, etc.), such diseases have
spread in irrigated areas, especially in the tropics (Eckolm,
1978; Euseby, 1979; Omo-Fadaka, 1977).

Before the construction of the dam on the Volta in Ghana,
the incidence of onchocercosis (a disease caused by worms
transmitted by fly bites) along the river was low. Today,
approximately half the river dwellers over 40 years old have
been blinded by onchocercosis, and the situation is becoming
worse (Johnson, 1972). In Cameroon, in villages near the
artificial lake created by the Bamendjin dam, 39 percent of the
population from 6 to 15 years old have been stricken with
malaria, while the incidence of malaria at Mendankwe, 28
kilometers from the lake, is only 1.9 percent. Onchocercosis
strikes 45 percent of the population in the villages near the
dam, as opposed to 3 percent at Mendankwe. Schistosomiasis
(bilharziasis), a disease caused by small worms transmitted by
snails, has infected about 200 million human beings and it
spreads rapidly near dams in the tropics (Eckolm, 1978).

Dams can also have disastrous consequences on the soil's
fertility. The best-known example is the Aswan (Taylor,

89

1970). The silt that used to fertilize the Nile valley each year is now held back by the dam. If "Egypt is a gift from the Nile," it is because of both the river's water and the silt it transports and deposits on the soil when the river recedes.

This silt used to be a complete natural fertilizer, containing a good many elements necessary for plant growth. It is now necessary to replace these nutrients with more costly chemical fertilizers that have less fertilizing value. Even more serious are the salt deposits that progressively sterilize the newly irrigated land because of insufficient drainage. According to the Egyptian minister of agriculture, more than half the irrigated land is threatened.

Certain dams provoke social and ecological disturbances. Some of the consequences of dam construction are that human populations may be displaced and fertile land covered with water, becoming unusable. The traditional means of food production may also be upset. For example, certain activities such as sardine fishing near the mouth of the Nile are almost certainly doomed to vanish.

It is possible to devise irrigation programs that don't produce these harmful effects. A few suggestions follow:

1. Villages should give small hydraulic systems priority over large projects (Thery, 1979). Operating small systems, which is much less expensive than large dams, does not present the same health, ecological, or social problems. Temporary wells or water gates are much less conducive to the development of parasite carriers. These small systems do not upset the ecological balance, nor is it necessary to displace people and completely change production systems.
2. In the cases where dams really would be useful, either for energy production or irrigation, it is often more advantageous to build several small dams instead of one large one.
3. Certain precautions may also be taken to limit parasite carriers (Dajoz, 1969):

   - stop the growth of aquatic vegetation along the dam's edges;
   - construct the overflow tank to avoid any steady leak which could serve as a place for parasite larvae to grow;
   - keep the riverbed downstream from the dam as clean and straight as possible, with no stagnant water;
   - offer health education for the people living near the dam.

Supplementary Readings for Question 6

> Are there ways to develop irrigation programs that are not harmful to the general health?

Diseases Transmitted by Water

Irrigated agriculture represents only 13 percent of the world's arable land, but crops produced on irrigated lands represent 34 percent of the world's total. The large amounts of development funds that have been channeled into irrigation projects are therefore understandable.

Yet, against the undeniable benefits these investments have brought, we must take into account the health problems that have resulted from inadequate planning of irrigation systems. Most developing countries still lack pure water, and waterborne or water-related diseases are endemic to wide areas. Only recently, however, have irrigation technicians begun to take these factors into consideration. (Many villagers near the Aswan dam still walk a mile for potable water.) The recommendations of health authorities for the zoning of the new agricultural workers' villages have frequently been disregarded at the planning stage. For example, health authorities advise leaving 300 meters between irrigation canals and inhabited areas, but these spaces are often filled with schools, public buildings, and even housing. Schoolchildren, the most prone to infection, use the canals for swimming or just cooling off.

Often, the distinction between waterborne and food-transmitted infections cannot be made, since food may be contaminated with pathogens contained in water and in turn serve as a vehicle for further infection. Lack of safe water in which to wash cooking and eating utensils can obviously play a part in spreading diseases.

The responsibility for bringing elementary health education to the villages has generally been left to local health and agricultural authorities. As yet, there appears to be no general health education system to inform workers and their families of new irrigation projects and the dangers that come with contaminated water. In developing countries, where increased crop yields have been considered of primary importance, health considerations are too often secondary, and diseases are apt to be considered part of the local way of life or death.

The most prevalent water-related afflictions are malaria, spread by 60 varieties of the anopheles mosquito, and onchocercosis, or river blindness, transmitted by small blackflies.

Among these, malaria has been the leading affliction, accounting for as many as 3 million deaths annually. There have been a number of successful malaria eradication programs over the years, including the campaign of the World Health Organization. Unfortunately, some of this effort has been negated by the impact of large irrigation and water-resource development projects that ultimately provide an ideal habitat for malaria-transmitting mosquitoes.

One example of what can happen is to be found in the Cukur and Antakya plains of Turkey, where a formerly swampy area was developed through irrigation and drainage for intensive farming of cereals, cotton, rice, vegetables, and citrus crops. Combined with rapid industrial growth in textiles, cement, and engineering, the agricultural development resulted in a large population influx of both seasonal farm workers and permanent industrial laborers.

Throughout the 1960s, a malaria eradication campaign had succeeded in reducing parasite incidence (API) from 10.3 to 0.002 per thousand inhabitants. The localities affected represented only 0.3 percent of the total area. In 1970, however, as a result of the growing influx of workers from eastern provinces where eradication programs were less advanced, a gradual resumption and spread of malaria transmissions became apparent. The proportion of affected localities rose to 18.4 percent in 1972 and 60 percent in 1976.

Excerpted from: *"Les projets d'irrigation ignorent les problèmes de santé" ("Diseases Reveal Lack of Planning in Water Schemes")* Cérès, *November-December 1979.*

Irrigation and Bilharziasis

The practice of irrigation, notably of rice paddies, has induced a renewed outbreak of disease in almost all the countries which have adopted it. In Egypt, for example, the rate of schistosomiasis infestation grew from 40 to 60 percent in the three years following the start of continuous irrigation.

The use of intermittent irrigation in Egypt and in the Philippines has produced spectacular agricultural yields. However, ways of maintaining the efficiency and economic advantages of irrigation (increased crop yields, increasing arable land surfaces, saving labor) without the accompanying financial, social, and health problems must be found. For instance, we could increase the use of rice varieties (such as *nadha*) which need less water without diminishing the yield; better still, we could practice crop rotation (alternating rice with other grains requiring less water) which would also destroy the schistosomiasis-host mollusks.

The evident upsurge of water-transmitted diseases in new development areas is finally beginning to attract some attention to the need for more careful and better coordinated planning of water-resource projects.

Excerpted from: *Euseby, C. "La bilharziose et le sous-développement: pour une approche globale du problème" ("Bilharziasis and Underdevelopment: a Global Approach to the Problem")* Tiers-Monde, *vol. XX, no. 80, October-December 1979, pp. 773-94.*

Irrigation and Schistosomiasis

The reservoirs and irrigation canals that turn lifeless lands into inviting human habitats create an ideal environment for the parasite-infested snails. Faced with a constantly mounting need for food and hydroelectric power, but short on money or the will to fight schistosomiasis, governments build new dams and irrigation systems, knowing full well that the disease will spread. Some 200 million people in at least 71 countries have already been afflicted, and there are more and more schistosomiasis victims each year.

Schistosomiasis primarily strikes the rural poor, which is one reason why so little has been done to halt its spread, to develop effective treatments, or even to chart its course. Unlike malaria, to which tremendous attention and resources have been devoted, schistosomiasis poses no threat to affluent urbanites. Only those who frequent infected canal or lake waters are likely to pick up the blood fluke, and only where sanitation is poor can the infection persist, since the fluke cannot reproduce unless it is returned to snail-infested water via human body wastes.

Because of their role in spreading schistosomiasis, many of Africa's major water developments in this century—including Lake Nasser in Egypt, Lake Volta in Ghana, the Gezira irrigation system in Sudan, and recent flood-rice projects in western Africa—have been called public-health disasters. Yet, in Africa and elsewhere, more such "seas of trouble" are being created every year.

The vast expansion of irrigated agriculture now being initiated throughout the Near East, southeast Asia, Africa, and Latin America poses a monumental public-health threat. The record of the past few decades of water-resource development is not encouraging. Dr. B. B. Waddy, who has studied the impact of dams on health in several countries, notes that national governments, private developers, and international aid agencies have all repeated avoidable mistakes "with monotonous regularity."

Excerpted from: *Eckolm, E. P. "La schistosomiase, une maladie des pauvres... et du développement" ("Schistosomiasis, a Disease of the Poor... and of Development")* Cérès, *January-February 1978, pp. 37-41.*

Destruction
of Disease-Carrying Mollusks

At present, the antischistosomiasis struggle is oriented toward the eradication of carrier mollusks. There are several ways to do this:

- using suitable grating to prevent penetration of mollusks into irrigated areas or by gathering mollusks to eliminate them;

- in rice paddies infested with schistosomiasis, not irrigating for two or three weeks between the germination and the flowering periods disturbs the mollusk cycle;
- maintaining the speed of water in the canals at greater than 0.30 meter per second avoids the proliferation of mollusks;
- destroying microflora through drainage or use of scythes can lead to the destruction of the mollusks.

Excerpted from: *"Mémento de l'adjoint technique des travaux ruraux" ("Notes from Rural Works Technical Assistant") Ministère de la Coopération, Paris, 1977, pp. 316-18: Mesures à prendre à la suite d'aménagements hydrauliques.*

Consequences of Large Dams

In industrialized countries, the introduction of technological methods requiring large capital investments has become a goal. The size of construction projects is linked to an increase in the Gross National Product (GNP).

Nonindustrialized countries are encouraged to follow the same path. But as the projects grow bigger and bolder every day, so do the problems fostered by them: rural and urban unemployment, malnutrition, and diseases such as sleeping sickness and malaria.

This is what Hughes and Hunter (1972) rightly called "development diseases" which are caused by a lack of ecological planning. The dam built on the Volta and the dams on the Aswan and the Kariba are examples of such ecological oversight (Milton and Farvar, 1973):

"The Aswan dam eliminated nutritive substances which, before, had furnished a regular supply of sardines; it caused some lakes to recede, thus reducing the available supply of fish protein; it allowed insecticides, herbicides, and molluscides to concentrate, thus causing the death of a great many fish. Moreover, the Nile delta, constantly eroded by the river current, is no longer protected by the sediment the river used to bring before the dam was built.

"In Egypt, the modern irrigation canals are ideal for the reproduction of carrier snails of parasite worms—schistosomes—from which people contact a debilitating disease, schistosomiasis. More than half the population of this country is stricken with schistosomiasis and much suffering has resulted. At the present time, prevention of this disease is all but impossible."

The dam on the Volta and the artificial Lake Volta are symbols of modern Ghana. It is true that the dam has solved many problems, but it has created others. The secondary effects of the dam have just begun to surface. Before its construction, there was a very low rate of onchocercosis along the Volta River . But at the present time, according to Johnson (1972):

"Perhaps half the river dwellers of the Volta over age 40 are blind, due to onchocercosis, and the situation is getting worse. The rise in cases of schistosomiasis is another serious secondary effect of the Volta dam. Before the creation of Volta Lake, the incidence of schistosomiasis along the river was low, but by the end of 1966, 10 percent of the children living along the river between the ages of 10 and 15 were stricken. At the end of 1968, the rate was nearly 100 percent; and in 1970, this statistic was virtually unchanged.

"Another problem was the relocation of displaced peasants. In addition to the difficulty of persuading them to move to a given location at a given time, there was also the problem of getting the peasants to accept and learn an entirely new kind of work and social system. This would require a total change in attitude, an acceptance of 'modern values' and 'modern ideas' about life. In the long run, the construction of the dam will mean a radical change in the life-style of many Ghanaians. Is it worth it?"

Excerpted from: *Omo-Fadaka, J. "Développement: la troisième voie" ("Development: the Third Way")* Environnement Africain, *vol. II, 4 and III, 1, November 1977.*

Some Unforeseen Consequences of the Nasser Dam

The most striking, and quite unexpected, consequence of the building of the Nasser dam has been the collapse of the Mediterranean sardine-fishing industry. The Mediterranean is poor in nutrients, except at the eastern end where the Nile used to discharge its rich burden of organic silt. The Egyptian sardine industry amounted to 18,000 tons, worth $7 million— sardines were almost half the total marine catch. Now the

Nasser dam holds back the silts, and today the sardine industry runs about 500 tons, while the export of fish products generally fell to half in the four years following the completion of the dam.

The loss of silt also means that the lower Nile Valley, once so fertile, now has to be treated with artificial fertilizer. The government, therefore, has to build fertilizer factories and divert some of the electric power created by the dam to run them. The dam is intended gradually to bring into cultivation an additional 2 million acres. However, there is an enormous loss of water by evaporation from the 200-mile-long Lake Nasser, behind the dam, and from the irrigation ditches—more than the whole amount supplied by the pre-existing dam. It is considered there will actually be less water than was available before, quite apart from that lost by seepage. True, the water will be where it is wanted, though only the alluvium along the river bank is fertile: away from the river the land is completely desert. Dr. A. A. Ahmed, a former technical consultant to the Egyptian Ministry of Public Works, has been quoted as saying that "evaporation losses appear to be so great as to make the High Dam of doubtful benefit, if not hazardous." Dr. Ahmed reckons that the whole of the Nile discharge could be lost by seepage during the first 20 years of its life, and about 70 percent during the next 10 years. Filling the Wadi Rayan would have been cheaper, he thinks, and just as effective.

But a still more serious consequence of this undertaking is the spread of the revolting disease known in Africa as bilharziasis, and elsewhere as schistosomiasis. The disease is caused by a blood fluke which is carried by snails but lays its eggs in man; the eggs are excreted into water, where they develop into larvae which enter snails. Here they develop into forked-tailed worms which attach themselves to people who enter the water; they bore through the skin and make for the liver, where they lay more eggs.

Now that malaria is largely under control, schistosomiasis has become the world's most widespread disease, afflicting an estimated 114 million people.

In Egypt the disease is already frighteningly common, owing to the general practice of excreting into the rivers and streams, and the lack of piped water. People also enter the streams either to bathe or wash, or to water animals, and become reinfected. It has been common since the time of the Pharaohs. Today it is reckoned that 70 percent of the population of Lower Egypt are affected: in some villages the rate is 100 percent. The life expectancy for women is 27 years, for men, 25. The rate at which the eggs are produced is fantastic. Dr. C. H. Barlow, who deliberately infected himself in the cause of science in 1944, produced 30,000 eggs a day. He became extremely ill and was only cured after a year and a half by means of a drug so unpleasant in its effects that most people refuse to complete the treatment.

The warm, slow-moving waters of irrigation ditches provide just the habitat that the host snails like, and favor the worst intestinal form of the disease; as irrigation spreads, so does schistosomiasis. Moreover, the ditches are kept filled year-round. Formerly, they dried in winter, and the cold tended to destroy the hosts. Dr. Henry van der Schalie considers that the spread of schistosomiasis may well cancel out all the benefits of this $1.3 billion undertaking.

Excerpted from: *Taylor, G. R.* The Doomsday Book, *Thames and Hudson Ltd., London, 1970, pp. 89-91.*

A Bihar Peasant Invents a Bamboo Tube Well

As has already been shown, construction of large dams for the purpose of irrigation can have adverse effects on the lives of those who use the water from the resultant lakes or irrigation ditches. It is known, however, that the availability of water for irrigation is an indispensable condition for increasing yields, especially with high-yield varieties of wheat. Thus, in India, the states of Punjab and Haryana very quickly put their undergound water sources to good use. However, this has not been the case in large sectors of the Ganges plain, in the east of Uttar Pradesh, and in Bihar. In spite of an abundance of water, Bihar had only 1,600 iron-tubed wells, as the result of a program that lasted from 1969 to 1973. The cost of the raw materials for these wells was exorbitant: 4,000 rupees per well, plus the same again for a diesel pump.

Unfortunately, simplified technology existing in Western Bengal had scarcely penetrated Bihar. In Bengal, wells could be built for 800 to 900 rupees from an iron stem fixed on iron rings, all wrapped in coco fiber string.

The first one to make full use of agricultural resources in Bihar was an individual peasant prompted by need. With four hectares to cultivate, Ram Prasad bought a pump despite the fact that he lacked a reliable water source. In the winter of 1968, a neighbor promised to give Prasad his used tube well. Based on this promise, he sowed several new types of crops. When the neighbor changed his mind, Prasad spent several sleepless nights wondering how to save his harvest from disaster. He knew about the use of coco fiber to make a filter/strainer. He decided to make a simplified tube well with 6-meter strips of bamboo adjusted on rings of iron, waterproofing the upper part of the tubes with old jute sacks coated with tar. All his friends and neighbors thought he was crazy, but after the second attempt, thanks to the sandy content of the local soil, the bamboo tubes held up when they were set in place.

The local development agent and the agricultural director of Prasad's district became enthusiastic about the procedure and encouraged the other growers to try it. They were impressed by its modest cost (250 rupees) as well as the apt use of local materials. It was possible for ten workers to build a tube well in one day with the help of the village blacksmith; 4,000 wells were made in four years.

The technical department of the State of Bihar objected to the bamboo well, saying it would be destroyed by air, water, ants, rodents, and soil pressure. However, when the drought began in 1972, the oldest of these wells had been in operation four years! An emergency plan for the building of 14,000 wells enabled nearly 100,000 hectares of arable land to benefit from irrigation. Similarly, a credit program was begun which made it possible for even the poorest peasants to rent diesel pumps mounted on wheels.

Excerpted from: Thery, D. *"Héritage et créativité du savoir écologique populaire comme facteurs de développement sous-utilisés"* (*"Heritage and Creativity of Popular Ecological Knowledge as Factors of Under-Utilized Development"*) Nouvelles de l'Écodéveloppement, no. 10, September 1979, pp. 8-31.

Question 7

Are the food-processing techniques of industrialized countries the most effective from an economic and nutritional standpoint?

Food processing in an industrialized country often means costly, polluting factories (see table 7–1) that employ little of the work force. These factories consume much energy, recyclable raw materials, and water. The concentration of factories, furthermore, necessitates expensive transportation and infrastructural supports.

It is no wonder processed food costs more. Increased costs are the result of preparation, packaging, and other processes which nutritionally deplete the final product more than they add to its value (Chonchol,1980).

Industrial processing techniques almost always cause food products to lose some nutritional value. When many foods are refined (grains, salt, sugar) or preserved through other modern methods (canning, freezing), a large part and in some cases all of the vitamins and minerals are lost. Grain foods such as white bread, white noodles, and white rice lose from 60 to 85 percent of their vitamins and from 50 to 60 percent of their minerals (see chart 4 and tables 7–2 and 7–3).

White sugar is composed of pure sucrose and no longer contains minerals or vitamins. Not only does it have no food value (aside from calories), but it is one of the main causes of heart disease, diabetes, and dental caries in industrialized countries (Aubert, 1983). Salt, another refined product, is very low in magnesium and other minerals. Equally controversial is the food industry's use of multiple chemical additives (colorings, preservatives, antioxidants, emulsifiers, and texture agents), since little is known about the long-term effects. Certain additives, nontoxic in themselves, reinforce the harmful effects of other chemical substances. For example, certain emulsifiers encourage the body's absorption of carcinogenic substances.

Table 7-1 Water pollution resulting from food-processing industries

Agricultural and food-processing industries	Sources of the principal wastes	Characteristics
Canned fruits and vegetables Potato industry	Cleaning, squeezing, blanching, and pressure cooking of fruits and vegetables	High MS content; gels and organic material dissolved; pH sometimes alkaline; starch
Meat processing and salting	Sheepfolds, slaughter-houses, treatment of entrails, condensers, fats and water from washing	High concentration in dissolved organic material and in suspension (blood, proteins), fats, NaCl
Food for livestock	By-products from centrifuge treatment, pressing, evaporation and residue from washing	Very high DBO*, only organic materials, odor solvents
Dairies	Dilutions from whole milk, skim milk, buttermilk, and serum	Very high concentration of dissolved organic materials, mainly protein, lactose, fats
Sugar refineries	Washing and transportation of sugar beets: diffusion, removal of scum, condensed evaporation, regeneration of ion exchangers	Very high concentration in dissolved organic matter and matter in suspension (sugars and protein)

Agricultural and food-processing industries	Sources of the principal wastes	Characteristics
Breweries and distilleries	Soaking and pressing the grain, residue from alcohol distillation, condensed evaporation	High content in dissolved organic matter containing sugar and fermented starch
Yeast plants	Residues of yeast filtration	High content in dry matter (especially organic) and in DBO*, high acidity
Vegetable oil and margarine industry	Extraction and refining	High fat and saline content; high acidity, very high DBO*
Dehydrated food and concentrates	Freeze drying and many other processes	Matter in suspension; diverse residues, high DBO* and coloration; many fats and oils present
Nonalcoholic drinks	Washing bottles, cleaning the floor and equipment, waste from syrup storage vats	High alkaline content, high content of substances in suspension and DBO*; detergents
Tanneries	Soaking, liming, dipping, dewooling, preserving the skins, tanning and drying baths	High content in dry matter, hardness, salt, sulfur, chrome, lime precipitate and DBO*
Starch works and glucose production	Condensed evaporations, syrup from final washing	High DBO* content and dissolved organic matter (in particular, starch and by-products)

*Demande biologique en oxygène = biological oxygen demand.

Excerpted from: Degremont, Sté, "Mémento technique de l'eau," Rueil-Malmaison, 1972.

Chart 4

Nutritional Consequences of Refining Wheat Flour

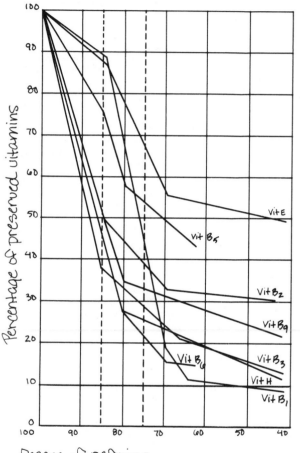

Degree of refining
Whole grain flour → Refined white flour

Excerpted from: Aykroyd, W.R. et Doughty,). "Le blé dans l'alimentation humaine" ("Wheat in the Human Diet"), L'Organisation des Nations Unies pour l'alimentation et l'agriculture, Rome, 1970.

Table 7-2   Nutritional value of potatoes in different
                  forms

	Baked potato	Frozen french fries	Dehydrated mashed potato	Potato chips
Calories	100	100	100	100
Weight (g)	139	145	27	17.50
% water	75.1	52.9	5.2	1.8
Protein	2.7	1.6	1.95	0.96
Sugars	22.6	15.3	23.0	8.8
Fat	0.14	3.8	0.18	7.0
Iron (mg)	0.76	0.8	0.49	0.35
Vitamin B_1 (mg)	0.11	0.06	0.06	0.035
Vitamin B_2 (mg)	0.05	0.01	0.018	0.008
Vitamin B_3 (mg)	1.86	1.16	1.46	0.87
Vitamin C (mg)	21	9	8.5	2.6

In relation to baked potatoes, chips contain, for the same amount of caloric content, 50 times more fat, 2 times less iron, 3 times less vitamin B_1, 6 times less vitamin B_2, 8 times less vitamin C.

Excerpted from: "Dietary Goals for the United States," Selected Committee on Nutrition and Human Needs, U.S. Senate, Washington, D.C., 1977.

Home food-processing methods are often superior to those in industry. For example:

● Whole grain bread and brown rice have a nutritive value that is far superior to that of white bread or white rice. They can be made from raw wheat or rice for a family or an entire village, with the help of simple and cheap facilities: stone-grinding mills and simple rice-hullers.
● Sugar from raw sugar cane (Indian *gur* or its Latin American equivalent *panella*) is 20 to 50 times richer in minerals and vitamins than refined white sugar; it can also be produced in small-scale business operations (see tables 7–4 and 7–5).

Table 7-3   Brown rice compared to other types of rice

	Composition of brown rice (per 100 g or 3½ oz)	Composition of other types of rice					
		White rice		Enriched white rice		Converted rice (enriched)	
Protein	7.5 g	6.7 g	90%	6.7 g	90%	7.4 g	99%
Minerals							
Calcium	32 mg	24 mg	75%	24 mg	75%	60 mg	190%
Phosphorus	221 mg	94 mg	43%	94 mg	43%	200 mg	90%
Iron	1.6 mg	0.8 mg	50%	2.9 mg	180%	2.9 mg	180%
Potassium	214 mg	92 mg	43%	92 mg	43%	150 mg	70%
Sodium	9 mg	5 mg	56%	5 mg	56%	9 mg	100%
Vitamins							
Thiamine	0.34 mg	0.07 mg	21%	0.44 mg	130%	0.44 mg	130%
Riboflavin	0.05 mg	0.03 mg	60%	0.03 mg	60%	0.03 mg	60%
Niacin	4.7 mg	1.6 mg	34%	3.5 mg	74%	3.5 mg	74%

Excerpted from: Moore Lappé, F. *Diet for a Small Planet,* revised edition, Ballantine, New York, 1978, p. 447.

Table 7-4	Comparison of nutritional value of refined and raw sugar	

	Per 100 grams of	
	Crystallized white sugar	Raw sugar
Sucrose	99.6 g	75 to 88 g
Glucose	0 g	2 to 9 g
Fructose	0 g	3 to 10 g
Water	0.05 g	2 to 4 g
Minerals	30 to 50 mg	1,500 to 2,800 mg
Potassium (K)	3 to 5 mg	600 to 1,000 mg
Magnesium (Mg)	0	60 to 130 mg
Calcium (Ca)	10 to 15 mg*	40 to 110 mg
Phosphorus (P)	0.3 mg	14 to 100 mg
Iron (Fe)	0.1 mg	4 to 40 mg

*This calcium comes for the most part from the lime added to the cane juice in the refining process.

Excerpted from: Beguin, Dr. M. H. "Aliments naturels, dents saines," Éd. de l'Étoile, La Chaux de Fonds, 1979.

● Preservation methods using lactic acid fermentation are in every way superior to modern techniques using cold or heat. Lactic acid fermentation can be done with easily acquired wooden barrels or stone jars; it uses no energy and, most remarkably, it increases the nutritive value of food (Aubert, 1979 and 1985). Here are several examples:

• When cabbage is made into sauerkraut, the lactic acid fermentation process is accompanied by an increase in the amount of vitamin C (through bacterial synthesis) and an improvement in digestibility.
• The sourdough used to leaven bread destroys the phytic acid in grains (which can inhibit the body's absorption of certain minerals).

Table 7-5   Comparison of small enterprise production (raw sugar) and industrial production (refined sugar) from cane sugar

| | Small enterprise raw sugar | | | Industrial white sugar | |
	Small workshop type Niger-Nigeria	Small workshop Panela, Colombia	Large workshop Panela, Colombia	Banfora refinery Upper Volta	Refinery projects in Nigeria
Capacity (tons of cane/day)	1.5	15	60	2,200	500
Annual production of sugar (tons)	7.5	225	900	2,700	6,750
Area of cane fields (ha)	1.5	45	180	3,900	1,500
Jobs involved in sugar manufacture	1.5	10	41	600	53
Number of jobs to produce 100 tons of sugar	200	44	46	22	8
Investment total (francs CFA)	200,000	5.5 million	29 million	10 billion	2.24 billion
Investment per job (francs CFA)	133,000	550,000	707,000	16.7 million	42.3 million

Excerpted from: BIT (Bureau International du Travail) "Technologies appropriées dans les industries de transformation alimentaire et de conservation.

• Soybeans, a food exceptionally rich in protein (about 40 percent), are difficult to digest, even after prolonged cooking. Since time immemorial, Asians have processed soybeans through fermentation in order to obtain food products that are more digestible, richer in protein and other nutrients, and better tasting. Some examples are tofu and soy sauces of China and Japan, and the tempeh of Indonesia. These products are not only easily digested and richer in vitamins than unfermented soybeans, but they also add variety to a low-meat diet. Also, tempeh contains vitamin B_{12}, highly valued because of its rarity in vegetables.

• West Africans make *soumbala*, a fermented product obtained from the seeds of a leguminous shrub, *Parkia biglibosa* (locust bean). Unfermented, the locust bean seeds are very hard and practically inedible. The traditional fermentation process yields a product that is high in protein (up to 50 percent), keeps well in tropical climates, and is an ingredient in many dishes.

• Traditional fermented grain-based beverages (beer, African kaffir beer, South American *chicha*, Russian *kvass*, Slavic *braga*, etc.) are also superior to beverages produced by the modern food-processing industry. Their small-scale production is simple and requires no costly material, and they are rich in protein, vitamins, and minerals. For example, kaffir beer contains vitamin B_{12}, which millet itself lacks. The alcohol content of these drinks is generally very low (1 to 4 percent), and, of course, they contain no chemical additives.

In developing countries, the food-processing industry should not follow the Western model. But cola beverage plants, industrial breweries, sugar refineries, and canneries are being built everywhere in the Third World. Most of their output is intended for domestic consumption. The sugar industry's rate of growth—to cite just one example—is rapid and particularly alarming. Outside of its caloric content, refined sugar's properties are all harmful to health. Public and private sector investments in sugar refineries and money spent on refined sugar by consumers could be used for the production and purchase of much more nutritious food.

It is important to stop or at least to slow down this trend and to develop less costly food-processing technology in these countries, so that food with a higher nutritive value will continue to be produced. Many traditional techniques can be perfected in order to reduce the time devoted to preparing food and still maintain food quality. A few examples of these techniques are the grinding and processing of grains, the making of *gari* from cassava, the brewing of beer from millet, and the making of palm wine (Fyot, 1973).

In industrial countries it can be noted that a small but growing segment of the population rejects many of the food-processing industry's products because of their harmful effects. People are replacing processed foods with products that have not been denatured (whole grains, lactic-acid fermented foods, fresh or dried fruits and vegetables) and which can often be made by small businesses.

The growing awareness is particularly noticeable in the most industrialized regions. The return to "natural" foods, far from being just a fad as some claim, is a reaction against food products that have become insipid and have lost a good part of their nutritional value.

Supplementary Readings
for Question 7

Are the food-processing techniques of industrialized countries the most effective from an economic and nutritional standpoint?

The Failure of Techniques
Imported from the West

In many developing countries, production for domestic markets is done with modern techniques imported from the West. These techniques are very costly in view of available resources, especially because the processing is patterned after industrialized countries where the goal is to raise the cost of the final product in relation to its initial agricultural value.

This type of food production establishes a market price beyond the buying power of the poorest economic groups and, at the same time, diminishes the food's nutritional content.

Excerpted from: Chonchol, J. "L'échec des solutions productivistes" ("The Failure of Productivity Solutions") Politique Aujourd'hui, no. 1-2, January-February 1980, pp. 61-70.

The Harmful Effects of Refined White Sugar

An example of this is seen in the harmful effects of refined white sugar. A comparison of industrial technology and traditional technology used in processing cane sugar shows that, from all points of view, traditional technology is preferable. It furnishes a much more nutritious product, raw sugar (Indian *gur* or Colombian *panella*), which can be made by tradespeople on a small-scale. The reduction in manpower brought about by industrial technology is more and more a disadvantage than an advantage in our age of widespread unemployment.

Making white sugar from the sugar beet is an entirely different problem, since it is impossible to extract sugar from the beet by small-scale techniques. But white sugar, whatever its source, should be eliminated or, at least, carefully controlled in our diets. The dangers it presents to health are many:

- Vitamin and mineral deficiencies: Sugar constitutes a great part of the caloric intake, and since there is a total absence of minerals and vitamins ("empty calories") in refined sugar, many deficiencies may result.
- Tooth decay: It is well known that sugar is the main cause of this. Dental caries are the main type of infection in developing countries and can precipitate a wide range of illnesses.
- Overweight and obesity: Sugar, like fat, leads to excess weight, for it contains empty calories in a concentrated form.
- Diabetes: It is proven that sugar is an indirect cause of diabetes, being a factor of obesity and excessive absorption of fats (many sugary foods—ice cream, pastry, chocolate—are rich in fats too). And obesity or simply being overweight are factors leading to diabetes. The direct role of sugar in the occurrence of diabetes (sugar causes a drastic rise in blood glucose levels) has not been determined.
- Cardiovascular diseases: When it is combined with saturated fats, sugar leads to cardiovascular diseases. The effect of sugar alone has not been determined.
- Cancer: Sugar is not in itself carcinogenic, but it tends to weaken the organism's natural defenses, primarily through notable vitamin deficiencies (vitamin A may act as a defense against certain forms of cancers).

Excerpted from: *Aubert, C.* L'assiette aux céréales (The Cereal Bowl) *Éd. Terre Vivante, Paris, 1983.*

Beneficial Changes through Fermentation

Fermentation greatly changes the composition of food. Certain substances are broken down while others are synthesized by active microorganisms. These phenomena are not well understood, but the following processes have been noted:

- Certain undesirable substances are destroyed, such as trypsin inhibitors, hemoaglutines, saponines, which are found in certain legumes, and phytic acid, found in grains.
- Many enzymes are synthesized by microorganisms (proteolases, amylases, lipases, cellulases, hemicellulases). These enzymes transform proteins into amino acids which are more easily assimilated and digested by the human body. For example, sauerkraut is easier to digest than nonfermented cabbage, and tamari and miso are easier to digest than soybeans.
- The fermentation process may also enhance vitamin synthesis. It has often been said that lacto-fermented products have a higher vitamin content, especially of vitamins B and C, than nonfermented ones (see chart 5). Researchers have discovered the presence of vitamin B_{12}, which is particularly rare in vegetarian diets, in soy-fermented preparations. This vitamin is synthesized by the microorganisms responsible for fermentation, since it is minimally present in raw soybeans (see table 7–6).

Excerpted from: *Aubert, C.* Une autre assiette (Another Plate) *Éd. Debard, Paris, 1979, p. 300.*

Fermentation Effects in Leguminous Plants

In 1943 British prisoners of war in a Japanese prison camp obtained some soybeans to add to their limited and deficient diet, consisting almost entirely of milled rice. It was recognized

Chart 5

Vitamin C Content in Fermenting Sauerkraut

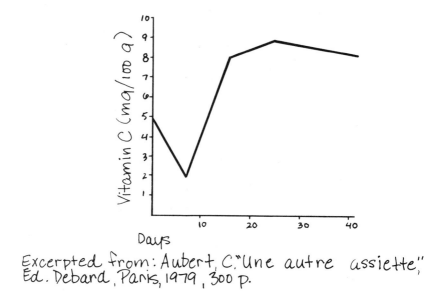

Excerpted from: Aubert, C."Une autre assiette"
Ed. Debard, Paris, 1979, 300 p.

Table 7-6   Vitamin content in soybeans and tempeh
(fermented soybeans)

Vitamin	Soybeans (mg/g)	Tempeh (mg/g)
Riboflavin	3	7
Pantothenate	4.6	3.3
Thiamine	10	4
Niacin	9	60
B_{12}	0.15 μg	5 μg

Excerpted from: Van Veen, A. C., and Steinkraus, K. H., "Nutritive Value and Wholesomeness of Fermented Food," *Journal of Agricultural and Food Chemistry*, vol. 18, no. 4, August 1970, p. 576.

that the high nutrient content of the beans would make them a valuable supplement to this diet. At first they were simply boiled, but in this form were found to be unpalatable and exceedingly indigestible; many men passed unaltered beans in their stools. Some Dutch prisoners suggested that the beans should be made into tempeh by the process followed in the East Indies and a makeshift plant for the purpose was rigged up in the camp. A culture of the necessary fungus was obtained from the withered petals of a hibiscus plant. Soaked dehusked beans were seeded with the fungus, placed on trays covered by sacking, and left for 48 hours to become a grayish rubbery mass, which was eaten after frying. The preparation was found to be crisp, brown, appetizing, and readily digestible and was "successfully used in treating protein and vitamin deficiencies."

This account comes from one particular prison camp, but soybeans were prepared for consumption in much the same way in a number of other camps, with similar results. Such experiences demonstrate the effect of fermentation on nutritive value more vividly than detailed laboratory analysis. First, the effect is "mechanical," i.e., all parts of the legume are fragmented so that they are easily reached by the digestive juices. Secondly, a large proportion of the protein is broken down into constituent amino acids which are readily absorbed and utilized, and it appears that the so-called trypsin inhibitor is destroyed. There may be some increase in nutrient content resulting from the growth of the fermenting organism itself, but no figures to show this have been found. The main effect of fermentation, whatever the fermenting agent used, is to make the nutrients present in the grain more fully available. It also leads to the formation of antioxidants which have a preservative action particularly valuable in tropical conditions.

Recent experiments with rats have shown that the proteins in tempeh have a higher biological value than those of unfermented soybean preparations. The Protein Efficiency Ratio (PER) of tempeh was found to be equivalent to that of skim milk powder. Prolonged feeding with unfermented soybean preparations produced hepatic injury in rats which did not occur in animals given tempeh.

Some observations on the nutritive value of the fermented preparation, *idli*, have been made in India. As a result of fermentation, there was an increase in choline, methionine, and folic acid content, but no vitamin B_{12} appeared. Feeding *idli* to rats on a high-fat, low-protein diet seemed to protect them from liver damage, and the fermented mixture had a greater regenerating effect on red blood cells than the same mixture before fermentation.

Excerpted from: *Aykroyd, W. R. and Doughty, J. "Legumes in Human Nutrition," FAO, Washington, D.C., 1974.*

Semi-Industrial Manufacture of Palm Wine

Palm wines, made in many countries of the intertropical forest zone, are produced from the natural fermentation of the sap of palm trees. The nature and quality of palm wine depend on the variety and location of the palm tree from which it comes, the point on which the tree is tapped, and other factors. Raphia wine, extracted from the raphia palm in Cameroon, has a characteristic taste unlike ordinary palm wine. However, all of these wines have in common the property of fermenting very rapidly. In 24 hours, they become undrinkable, even under a controlled temperature.

Raphia palms are cultivated bordering the small river channels in the lower regions. Before it bears fruit, a crack is made at the base of the raphia tree. The sap flows out drop by drop into half a hollowed-out gourd at the rate of about two liters per tree per day. The gathering takes place twice a day: in the evening around 6 P.M. (the "winegrower" stores the sap overnight in 2- to 5-liter gourds) and in the morning between 5 and 7 A.M. when the sap is mixed with that of the previous evening. The wine is distributed to the villages and consumed or sold that very day in local markets.

The prices of these beverages vary greatly—they can even triple from one day to the next as a function of supply and demand. The average price of a winegrower's product varies each year between 14 and 20 F *CFA* per liter (1 F *CFA* equals 0.02 FF). A substantial amount of the wine is transported to neighboring urban centers, often by bicycle. There the wine is resold in the market once or twice and finally delivered to the consumer at a price of 30 to 40 F *CFA* per liter.

Collecting the sap in ordinary calabash gourds is a natural way of providing it with yeast and bacteria—both the culture medium and temperature conditions are ideal. In a few hours, the sap is fully fermented. In six hours the sugar is practically gone, as lactic and acetic acids replace the yeast.

Because of the popularity of the beverage, it was natural to try to control fermentation in order to keep the wine longer without affecting its quality. This would also make it possible to supply wine to the nonproductive regions which do not have fresh wine. The home market is, indeed, quite large—in 1969–1970 the Republic of Cameroon consumed nearly 405 million liters of drinks made locally or imported, of which palm wine represented 280 million liters.

Palm wine is produced on a large economic scale in Cameroon, as well as in many countries along the Gulf of Guinea and in Central Africa. The stabilization of palm wine would prevent many losses due to rapid fermentation and would provide a drink of consistent quality which could be easily marketed. The beverage would also be more bacteria-free without losing its nutrients. Some analytical work was done at ORSTOM by Mr. Bergeret and Mr. Périssé and also by Mr. Adriaens, who was in charge of the Laboratory of Chemical Research in Brussels. Their research led to the conclusion that fresh palm wine is a good source of vitamin C (120 to 250 milligrams of ascorbic acid per liter) and a modest source of vitamin B_1 (0.06 to 0.07 milligram per liter of riboflavin). The fermented wine contains no methanol, aldehydes, or ketones and seems to be completely nontoxic.

Once stabilized, this drink could sell quite well both at home and abroad if seriously marketed. This is particularly true of Europe, where exotic products have been very successful with diverse population groups. Because of these observations, the SATEC mission, which promotes small and average-size businesses in Cameroon, is working with the Ministry for Industrial Development to explore the technical possibilities of stabilizing raphia wine through a pasteurization process.

The principle consists of destroying, as thoroughly as possible, the bacterial flora present in the raw juice. Many procedures had to be tested before arriving at a satisfactory solution. In the course of treatment, the wine undergoes a total de-aeration which removes its sparkling flavor. This necessitates a second, controlled fermentation to restore the gas, and then a second pasteurization. The results are excellent. The treated wine can be kept for more than a year without change. Furthermore, analyses done at the Pasteur Institute show that the wine obtained is much safer for consumption. The pasteurized palm wine has the following properties:

pH = 3.9
Total acidity = 2.49 grams/liter
Reducible sugars in glucose = 21 grams/liter
SO/2 = 18 milligrams/liter

This experiment involving the commercial preparation of a traditional drink is unique and should spread rapidly. Countries such as Nigeria and Zaire have already shown interest in the procedure. Although more research will undoubtedly be necessary to improve the treatment process, it is now clear that it is rich in technical and commercial possibilities. It is also possible that mobile stabilization units for palm wine will one day be created to make use of older plantation stock chopped down to make room for new trees.

Excerpted from: *Fyot, R. "La valorisation industrielle d'une boisson traditionnelle: le vin de palme pasteurisé" ("Industrial Stabilization of a Traditional Drink: Pasteurized Palm Wine")* Techniques et Développement, *July-August 1973, pp. 28-29.*

═══════ Question 8 ═══════

Are food imports justified from a nutritional
standpoint?

Developing countries that were once self-sufficient, as
were all countries before the industrial revolution, are now
importing more and more food products. These imports aim, on
the one hand, to fill the deficit in primary food products
(principally grains). The chief causes of this deficit are the
upsetting of the demographic balance and, more importantly,
the increase in export crop production.

On the other hand, there has been an increasing demand
for Western food products (bread, sugar, beverages, milk
products, Western fruits and vegetables). This attraction to
the Western food model arises, in part, from multinational
firms' advertising, mainly in cities, and has resulted in an
increase in food imports (Dupin, 1975).

However, importation of primary food products brings no
long-term solution. When there is a bad harvest, it seems that
importation is the only answer to the threatening situation.
But self-sufficiency in obtaining staple foods is the only goal
that makes sense. Turning to imports presents several problems: it fosters dependence on a foreign country, storage and
preservation are difficult, domestic currency leaves the country, and incentives for producing domestic food crops decline.

In the case of grain crops, self-sufficiency could be at-
tained by restoring domestic food crops to their proper place in
development programs. As for protein deficiency, it results

more from poor handling of local resources than from a real deficit. A judicious use of vegetable protein, notably legumes cultivated in association with grains, would help to improve the protein levels considerably without increasing the land needed.

With respect to infant health, it is known that imported powdered milk can be disastrous to a baby's health when it replaces breast feeding. Human milk is perfectly adapted to the physiological needs of the infant and provides antibodies that increase resistance to infections. The child, moreover, stands the best chance of getting an uncontaminated, nutritionally complete food for free. Powdered milk is inferior to breast milk in nutritive value and, like patented baby formulas, is often prepared under deplorable hygienic conditions in developing countries or is overdiluted when money is scarce.

In the Third World, powdered milk is undeniably associated with many infant deaths. At the very least, abandonment of breast feeding is wasteful economically, yet it helps make multinational firms that manufacture baby formulas richer.

In Chile, the percentage of breast-fed babies has fallen in eight years from 95 to 6 percent; in Mexico from 98 to 40 percent; in Singapore from 77 to 5 percent (Strahm, 1977).

For people of all ages, the importation of processed food products may have a negative effect on nutrition. The majority of imported products—white flour, white sugar, artificial drinks, canned goods—are often nutritionally inferior to local products. Several studies have shown that before the importation of foreign products became widespread and before the effects of urbanization and the population explosion were felt, traditional diets kept people in good health. When Western diets were adopted, the general state of health in developing countries began to deteriorate (Mackay, 1959).

The eating habits in industrial countries may not be a good example for developing countries to follow. The higher life expectancy in industrial countries is explained more in terms of hygienic progress and lower infant mortality than by an improvement in diet. In fact, the growing frequency of "civilization" diseases (cancer, heart disease, diabetes, etc.) is troubling, and it should be noted that these diseases are striking younger and younger.

For this reason, industrialized countries are beginning to question their eating habits. We should draw from our ancestors' wisdom and knowledge which preserved human health for thousands of years instead of encouraging the present eating habits that have led to increased incidence of degenerative diseases (Sallenave, 1959; Shneour, 1975). Furthermore, emulation of the Western diet by developing countries should be discouraged as well (Selected Committee on Nutrition and Human Needs, U.S. Senate, 1977).

Supplementary Readings for Question 8

> Are food imports justified from a nutritional standpoint?

Importation and Exportation of Protein Foods by Sahel

In the Sahel during the drought the amount of protein in exported foods (mainly in the form of peanut cakes) was always much greater than that contained in imported foods. At the height of the drought from 1971 to 1973, the eight countries that were most affected (Mali, Ethiopia, Upper Volta, Mauritania, Nigeria, Senegal, Sudan, and Chad) exported, in spite of their low crop yields, two to five times more protein drawn from their earth than they imported in the form of cereals (see table 8–1).

Excerpted from: *Marloie, M. "L'abondance mal gérée" Le Monde Diplomatique, no. 314, May 1980, p. 14.*

The Western Feeding Model

The Western feeding model has spread throughout the Third World with the help of multinational firms. The power of advertising has also played an important role. In all the countries which we call "developing," ads for Coca-Cola can be

Table 8-1

	Protein (thousands of tons)		
	1971	1972	1973
In net cereal imports	79	74	103
In net peanut exports			
oil cakes	186	307	183
nuts	66	58	48
Total exports	252	365	231

found. Even in the smallest grocery stores and village shops, it is possible to find ads for cigarettes or for Nestle's products.

In 1972, General Foods Corporation spent $125 million for advertising alone in the United States and abroad, a sum quite a bit larger than the World Health Organization's budget for the same year, which was $82 million. As a rule, large multinational firms in the food industry have net holdings which are higher than the gross national products of the developing countries in which they set up operations.

Clever advertising has persuaded many women that "Milk that comes in a box at the drugstore is better than mother's milk." These women believe that because a box of milk is very expensive, it must be good. Or because it is imported from a rich country, it is prestigious. Or because it is sold in a pharmacy by people wearing white coats, it is better for the baby's health.

A bottle feeding using packaged milk can be catastrophic, however, in regions where the majority of women are illiterate and do not know the basic elements of hygiene. Even those that do know them often have difficulty applying them because they live in primitive dwellings without running water or refrigerators.

Exacerbating the problem are Third World business leaders who have often studied in Europe, the United States, or Canada and are inclined to adopt foreign methods perhaps unconsciously. It is understandable that these civil servants, engineers, and doctors might want to continue consuming the Western foods and drinks they have grown to like. But those whose social status is high—from village school teachers to heads of state—are carefully observed by those who live around them. How they eat (or dress or furnish their homes) gives those who surround them a certain image of what is good. Relatives not so well off, servants, and co-workers relate social success with eating habits and try to imitate them.

One sign of social success that is spreading throughout the developing world is the consumption of imported whiskey and other alcoholic beverages. If you walk through the populated neighborhoods of Abidjan, Accra, or Kinshasa, you will see countless bars and restaurants that serve wines and aperitifs. Many companies make large profits importing and distributing these drinks. They have built up the market through clever advertising, but the "trademark" of approval was first given by the upper class, the elite.

Excerpted from: *Dupin, H. "Le modèle alimentaire occidental" ("The Western Food Model")* Jeune Afrique, *Dossier Bis "La crise alimentaire mondiale," January-June 1975, pp. 58-60.*

Dangers of Bottle Feeding

For several years, the consumption of "artificial" food for nursing children has grown rapidly in the Third World. More and more women, perfectly capable of breast feeding, have stopped doing so because they have been led to believe that bottle feeding is more modern or better for the baby. A first consequence, economically speaking, is the loss of a "raw material" that is immediately usable and of unsurpassed quality: mother's milk. According to Alan Berg, assistant director for nutrition of the World Bank, the loss incurred by developing nations is estimated at three-quarters of a billion dollars per year for nonutilization of mother's milk.

To nourish her baby properly with a bottle, a mother must rigorously follow rules of hygiene: the bottle must always be clean, the water must be boiled, hands must be carefully washed, exact measurements of powder must be used. As a rule, these conditions are impossible to achieve in the Third World except for a thin layer of Westernized people. When the only water available is that of a stagnant pond or public fountain, when there is only one pot in which to cook the family's meal, when the housing situation precludes cleanliness, bottle feeding is a certain carrier of infection.

This is why a great many bottle-fed babies contract diarrhea and diseases brought on by malnutrition—marasmus or kwashiorkor. Surveys taken in Chile, Jamaica, and Galilee all reach the same conclusion: the infant mortality rate due to digestive infections is two to three times higher in bottle-fed children than in those who are breast-fed (Vargas, 1976).

Excerpted from: *Vargas, F. de "Lait en poudre et techniques de vente" ("Bottle-Feeding")* Le Monde Diplomatique, *July 1976, p. 6.*

The Disappearance of Breast Feeding

Switching to bottle feeding, which has been urged by advertising campaigns, is an aberration by economic as well as health and nutrition criteria. In the space of two decades, the food industry's intense advertising has led to millions of women abandoning breast feeding for the bottle.

In Chile, the percentage of breast-fed babies (up to 13 months old) dropped from 95 percent to 6 percent in eight years. In Mexico, the percentage (for babies up to 6 months) fell from 98 percent to 40 percent; in the Philippines (up to 12 months) from 63 percent to 43 percent; in Singapore (up to 3 months) from 77 percent to 5 percent (Strahm, 1977).

From an economic point of view, the disappearance of breast feeding in Chile represents an annual loss equivalent to the milk of 32,000 cows. In Western Europe, the cost of artificial food for a nursing baby three months old is equivalent to about 2 percent of a worker's salary. In Indonesia it is equivalent to 19 percent of the official minimum wage; in India, 23 percent; in Nigeria, 30 percent; in Pakistan, Egypt, and in many other countries, up to 40 percent.

The change from breast feeding to the bottle is economic and medical nonsense. It is senseless to pay a high price for a product of lesser quality which carries enormous risks instead of using a product of unequalled quality (mother's milk), that requires no complicated explanations, and is also free. The loss for underdeveloped countries caused by the purchase of powdered milk is estimated at several billion dollars.

Chart 6

Decline in Breast Feeding due to
Powdered Milk Advertisement

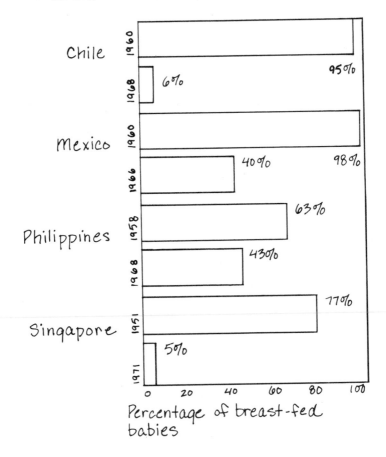

Percentage of breast-fed
babies

In spite of the exorbitant cost, many lower-class mothers in the Third World think they should use the bottle. They solve the problem by diluting the milk; the box, intended to last eight days, has to last for several weeks. Add to this poor hygiene, and the results are undernourishment, stomach and intestinal illnesses, long-lasting aftereffects, and a rise in the infant mortality rate.

The problem of bottle feeding was brought to light in the pamphlet "The Baby Killer" published by "War on Want" in 1974. The pamphlet severely criticized the advertising practices of the manufacturers of powdered milk, especially Nestle's. The company tried to sue a group in Berne who published the pamphlet in German under the title "Nestle's Kills Babies." The group was given a small fine, but the decision itself included this sentence: "Proof has been established that improper use of powdered milk can cause the death or serious illness of small children." This statement was supported primarily by declarations from the World Conference on Food (1974) and by several resolutions from the World Health Organization. Powdered milk is only one example of the absurdity of selling goods that do not satisfy the fundamental needs of the Third World population.*

Editor's note: A seven-year boycott against Nestle's products was ended in early 1984 when the American Infant Formula Action Coalition reached an accord with Nestle's. The accord hinged on the Swiss-based company's acceptance of four points. The company agreed to: (1) curtail promotional supplies of free infant formula to hospitals or health centers in developing countries, (2) stop providing material favors to doctors in exchange for promoting the formula, (3) place warning labels on the packages, and (4) include warnings of hazards of formula-feeding in its promotional literature.

Excerpted from: *Strahm, R. H. "Pourquoi sont-ils si pauvres?"* *("Why Are They So Poor?")* A la Baconnière/La Déclaration de Berne, *Neuchâtel, 1977, p. 147.*

Rice and Bread for Cities

The living conditions in a city make people look for grain foods that are inexpensive and as easy to prepare as possible. We know the choices: rice and bread. Food surveys taken in the urban environment leave no doubt about these preferences. Governments have often subsidized rice and wheat imports to make them accessible to the greatest number. The relatively small urban population (in Africa), as well as the relatively favorable exchange terms between agricultural exports and food imports, made this type of policy possible.

In 1975, millet, corn, and sorghum represented no more than one-tenth of the cereal consumption in Dakar. In other large Sahelian cities, however, consumption of these was 50 percent or more for all cereals consumed. And millet, corn, and sorghum still represent close to 100 percent of the total cereals consumed in rural zones.

Excerpted from: *Labonne, M. "Le déficit céréalier—D'où vient-il? Qui frappera-t-il? Quelle politique adopter?" ("The Grain Deficit— Where Does It Come From? Where Will It Strike Next? What Policy to Adopt?")* Afrique Agriculture, no. 50, October 1979, pp. 24-25.

The Passion for Imported Food

The passion for imported food is well demonstrated in the case of Nigerians who are generally quite conservative in their eating habits, but are currently eating more and more imported foods (for example, bread, cola, sugar, and others of this type).

Bread, a prestigious food, both drains a nation's financial resources and empties the peasants' purses—they now sell their products to have enough money to buy bread. Soft drinks are even worse. They are basically nothing but sugar, water, and colorings. In place of palm wine, villagers are adopting this type of drink more and more, especially at parties and receptions. The traditional bitter taste has been supplanted by a sugary taste and all the dangers that go with it.

As migration toward population centers continues, education improves, and the economy expands, there is a growing demand for all kinds of imported ready-made products. Urbanized villagers return to the village and sing the praises of prestigious sugared food, while advertising only makes matters worse.

It is possible in some cases for families to stock up on products because they keep well, resulting in better nutrition. But in most cases, nutrition suffers since, through ignorance, good fresh foods are sacrificed for less nutritious canned foods.

Excerpted from: *Oke, O. L. "La transformation traditionnelle des aliments au Nigeria" ("Traditional Food Processing in Nigeria")* Environnement Africain, vol. III, 3-4, no. 11-12, 1979.

Nutrition and Physical Degeneration

Observations have shown that populations who keep their traditional ways of eating have sound physical development and very few cavities. The opposite is true of "modern" individuals who have adopted Western eating habits: they have bone deformities, dental cavities, and many other pathological symptoms (Mackay, 1959).

The clinical findings of W. A. Price show that enormous differences exist between isolated peoples and modern peoples. A comparison of these groups shows that isolated peoples maintain a strong immunity to a great number of our medical conditions as long as they remain sufficiently isolated and live according to the "accumulated wisdom" of their tribes.

On the other hand, when isolated groups adopt the habits of our civilization, they rapidly lose the group's immunity. This basic difference between the isolated and the modernized is found everywhere in spite of differences in race, latitude, altitude, temperature, and climate.

The comparison further shows that, regardless of racial background, the great majority of subjects among isolated people have the following characteristics:

1. A robust quality, combined with a sound physical development.
2. Deformities and signs of degeneration are rare. This includes:

   - rarity of bone malformations: 3 to 8 percent of subjects.
   - few cavities: on the average, 1 percent of all teeth showed some decay.

3. Absence of obstetrical complications and ease of breast feeding, which is generally abundant and long-lasting.
4. Low death rate; rarity of tuberculosis, rheumatoid arthritis, cardiac problems, internal organ conditions, and malignant tumors.
5. Strong vitality with resistance to stress and efficiency at work.
6. Solid character; rarity of antisocial characteristics and criminal tendencies.

The modernized group, having come in contact with civilization, more frequently exhibits the following:

1. Weak and uncoordinated individuals.
2. Signs of degeneration, in particular:

    • bone deformities (25 to 83 percent), including narrow pelvis, tight thorax, foot deformities.
    • dental cavities (averages of 30 percent).
    • maxillofacial anomalies.

3. In certain cases, lowering of fertility, difficult pregnancies or births, and difficult nursing (breast feeding).
4. Higher death rate, due in particular to pulmonary tuberculosis and rheumatoid arthritis.
5. Loss of energy and moral values with a feeling of discouragement about life.

The primary orientation of Price's work is the important role of nutrition in maintaining physical health. In a painstaking analysis of his observations, Price discovered that one factor always varies when an individual moves from an isolated group to its modern racial counterpart: the diet. Specifically, replacing a natural diet (traditional foods) with civilization's industrialized food (white flour, refined sugar, canned foods, vegetable fats, polished rice, tea, coffee, chocolate) results in the characteristics listed above.

Among the most clear-cut cases is Switzerland. In the high valleys of this country, environmental factors are almost identical from one area and population group to another, except for food. In Vissoie and Ayer, two villages which are separated by several hours walk, clothing, houses, livestock, culture, and customs are exactly the same. But in Ayer, an isolated village, the inhabitants consume products made locally; in Vissoie, which is linked to the outside world by a road, peasants sell their rye and high-quality milk products and eat modern food. Signs of physical degeneration among the people of Vissoie are beginning to appear.

The importance of diet can often be seen through statistical trends. Let's look at one case history. Indians and Alaskan Eskimos can, in actuality, be subdivided into three distinct groups. Some are totally isolated and eat indigenous food. Others live in the immediate proximity of outposts of the

Hudson Bay Company and adopt modern food. Others are in the intermediate zone and frequently visit the outposts and, due to this fact, have a mixed diet. Signs of degeneration increase progressively from the isolated zone to the modern zone, as the percentages of cavities show:

Isolated Eskimos: 0.09 percent
Mixed Eskimos: 4 to 18 percent
Modern Eskimos: 31 percent

Isolated Indians: 0.16 percent
Mixed Indians: 14 to 17 percent
Modern Indians: 21.5 percent

Excerpted from: *Mackay, Dr. F. "Étude analytique et critique de l'oeuvre de W. A. Price (Thèse de doctorat)" ("Analytical and Critical Study of W. A. Price's Work [Doctoral Thesis]")* L'Alimentation Normale, *no. 21-22, AFRAN, Paris, 1959.*

Traditional Food and the Health of the Otomi Indians

Modern scientific methods are not always advantageous to a primitive people. In 1946 an extensive report was published by a joint team from the Rockefeller Foundation and the Mexican Government School of Hygiene, headed by Dr. Richmond K. Anderson, on the nutritional status and food habits of the Otomi Indians in the Mezquital Valley of Mexico. The Mezquital Valley lies 60 to 120 miles north of Mexico City astride the Pan-American Highway. The altitude of this arid, high plateau region is about 6,500 feet (2,000 meters) and good crops are hard to obtain. Maize and beans are staple foods. Pulque, the potent fermented drink made from the juice of the century plant, is important to both the economy and the nutrition of the Otomis.

In 1941 the Otomi Indians who populated the valley still clung to native customs in spite of the influence of the Spanish conquistadores of the early sixteenth century. Though many understood Spanish, most continued to use primarily the Otomi language. Most of the Otomis lived in small, one-room, dirt-floored huts that leaked badly when it rained. Clothing was meager, rarely washed, and passed on from parents to children. Louse infestation was universal because of poverty and scarcity of water, which had to be brought up with great effort from a few deep wells. Sanitary facilities and medical care were practically nonexistent.

Economically and culturally the Mezquital Valley was the most depressed region of Mexico. Yet the Otomi Indians made excellent use of the meager food resources available to them. Every edible plant was used as food, including many cacti. The Otomis also consumed a variety of worms and insects, which they ate with relish. By these means they maintained a diet of considerable variety and nutritional value. Some of the "weeds" the Otomis used as food proved on analysis to be nutritious and excellent sources of minerals, vitamins, and protein. Children were breast-fed, sometimes for several years, and the investigators reported that it was not unusual for a woman to have several children nursing at the same time. Since water was unsafe and hard to obtain, pulque was drunk in huge quantities by almost everyone, including babies and small children. Some of the men claimed that it served as a substitute for meat and that they were unable to work without it.

Because of the extreme aridity of the region, malaria was almost unknown in the Mezquital Valley. Considering the fact that the Otomi Indians practiced no dental hygiene, their teeth were remarkably good; nearly 50 percent of adult males had perfect teeth. Pronounced clinical nutritional deficiency was uncommon. Blood studies revealed values that compared favorably with those encountered elsewhere. The investigators ended their extraordinary report with the conclusion that the Otomi Indians had through many centuries developed a way of life and food habits that were well adapted to the hostile and barren land they occupied, and that it would be a mistake to attempt to change these habits until their economic and social conditions could be improved.

Excerpted from: Shneour, E. The Malnourished Mind, *Doubleday,* *New York, 1974, pp. 98-100.*

Nutrition and Disease Resistance in the People of Tonkin

Another example of the rewards of maintaining traditional eating habits is seen in the people of Tonkin, Vietnam.

In 1930, the railroad from Hanoi to Haiphong was not operating due to several dikes that had ruptured. These two cities are 110 kilometers apart, and people frequently went from one to the other by rickshaw. Preparation for the trip usually took place as follows:

A strong young rickshaw puller in Hanoi was hailed in the street and told the departure time. He let one of his friends know, and they both slept for two or three hours before departure. At the agreed hour, around 8 o'clock in the evening, the two runners came by with their rickshaw, and the trip began. It lasted all night, at an average speed of 10 to 12 kilometers an hour, one puller between the carriage shafts and the other in back.

Approximately every two hours, the pullers stopped in a village where they drank tea, ate a light bouillon (*pho*), rested for 5 to 10 minutes, and started up again. In the morning, they arrived in Haiphong, having covered 110 kilometers at a constant run. The runners rested during the day and generally left the same evening to return with more travelers to Hanoi.

This 110-kilometer trip in one night seemed absolutely normal to the Vietnamese. Yet I think that few European athletes could routinely run such a distance. This shows that the Vietnamese diet, based on polished rice and *nuoc-nam*, and including spiced herbs, fish, and meat in small quantities, natural sugar, and light tea, maintains a perfect balance in the body in spite of the hot climate and very hard physical labor.

Excerpted from: *Sallenave, P. "Cuisine et vitalité au Viet-Nam"* *("Cuisine and Vitality in Viet-Nam")* L'Alimentation Normale, *no. 21-22, AFRAN, Paris, 1959.*

═══════ Question 9 ═══════

Are there simple, inexpensive means to combat protein deficiencies?

Protein deficiency, a major problem in developing countries, is one of the most serious consequences of malnutrition. It appears in children as kwashiorkor which, even if the child survives, can do permanent damage (stunted growth, incomplete development of intellectual faculties, etc.). Protein deficiency also lowers resistance, so infectious diseases, that in themselves are benign (measles, chicken pox, intestinal diseases), can become mortal.

Increased animal protein in the diet (meat, fish, milk and dairy products, eggs) is the usual solution to this problem. But this is hardly an economical solution since turning of vegetable protein into animal protein is a very inefficient process. Depending on the type of production, three to ten kilograms of vegetable protein are required to manufacture one kilogram of animal protein.

When animals are fed products that humans do not eat (forage, various by-products), raising livestock becomes an appropriate and profitable way to make use of these products. But with intensive modern methods, animals are more often fed grains (corn, wheat, barley, oats), tubers (cassava, sweet potatoes, yams), or legumes (soybeans, peas, peanuts) which people can consume directly. Under these conditions the waste is obvious. It is also intolerable in a world where hundreds of millions of people have their calories rationed and receive insufficient protein. In the United States, almost 90 percent of grain production is used to feed animals. Thailand exports millions of tons of cassava to Europe where it is used to feed pigs.

Nonetheless, vegetable protein has been a major protein source for a great many people who consume only small amounts of animal protein. Vegetable protein is generally considered inferior to animal protein because it is low in certain essential amino acids. However, a judicious combination of vegetable proteins that contain complementary amino acids yields a protein very close in quality to animal protein. The most interesting and best-known example of this is the association of grains and legumes, the latter having the essential amino acid (most notably lysine) lacking in grains.

Vegetable protein sources are numerous. Whole grains (unrefined) contain 8 to 15 percent protein. In certain developing countries, grains provide more than half the protein supply. In these countries, grain refinement, which eliminates a good part of the protein, has particularly serious consequences. Legumes are the richest plant source of protein. Most of them (dried beans, peas, lentils, peanuts) contain 22 to 25 percent protein; others (soybeans, winged beans) contain up to 40 percent (Lozano, 1979). Nuts (walnuts, almonds, hazelnuts, pistachios) contain 13 to 20 percent protein, and seaweed as well as certain aquatic plants (water hyacinth) are also excellent protein sources (Fox, 1973).

Simple processes can improve the quality of vegetable protein as well as facilitate its assimilation in the human body. A few of these techniques follow:

- Combining complementary vegetable proteins renders the maximum amount of protein available. Combining grains and legumes, the most widespread association, is usually done at a ratio of 70 to 80 percent grain to 20 to 30 percent legume (Moore Lappé, 1976).
- The sprouting of grains is accompanied by a synthesis of essential amino acids. After six days of sprouting, wheat may contain up to twice as much lysine as before. Because lysine is the limiting amino acid in wheat, this process, widely used in the Middle East for making bulgur, has many beneficial effects.
- Lactic acid fermentation, especially of legumes, frees up some of the protein's amino acids and increases the amount of methionine (an indispensable amino acid) in grains.

Sprouting and fermentation make protein assimilation (especially of legume protein) more easy (see question 7).

The major part of small children's protein needs can be met with vegetable sources. The transition from breast feeding to food based on grains can be done without difficulty as long as weaning is neither too abrupt nor too early. Grains and legumes should be introduced gradually and properly prepared through slow cooking and/or toasting.

Supplementary Readings for Question 9

Are there simple, inexpensive means to combat protein deficiencies?

Vegetable Protein to Close the Food Gap

Legumes have been part of man's diet for a very long time. The discovery of seeds in the ruins of ancient Mexican and Egyptian civilizations has proven this. Inhabitants of these regions selected and cultivated wild plants and vegetables for thousands of years.

Out of the 13,000 known native legume species, only 10 to 12 are currently consumed on a regular basis. They are now of comparatively little economic importance (except for soybeans and peanuts, which have become commercial crops instead of subsistence crops). But they play an important part in the daily diets of many countries of the intertropical zone and, in particular, in African countries where the average consumption according to diet surveys is from 40 to 50 grams of legumes daily per person. This consumption varies largely from one region to another as a function of dietary habits, climatic conditions, and availability of other commodities (cereals) during different periods of the year (Lozano, 1979).

According to a recent report of the Food and Agriculture Organization (FAO), the amount of cultivated land area for all developing countries has increased only 10 percent in the past 20 years while the quantity of available legumes has not grown at all. In Africa, legumes production has not paralleled the rise in total cultivated area; in fact, legume crop yields as a whole are constantly dropping. In traditional farming systems, farmers are now putting most of their efforts into the most productive and financially rewarding crops (export crops).

Moreover, legumes, which are more difficult to store than cereals, undergo even greater losses after the harvest (primarily due to weevil infestation). Yet, legumes such as cowpea, horse grain, earth pea, pigeon pea, and dry beans are still very popular in Africa. Because of their high protein content (20 to 30 percent), they are an ideal complement to a diet based on cereals. For a small cost, they improve protein quality and balance amino acids in the recommended daily grain allowance by increasing lysine, threonine, and tryptophan content. They also contain substantial amounts of important minerals such as calcium and iron (100 milligrams of calcium and 7 milligrams of iron per 100 grams, on the average). Horse grain (a type of bean) contains 90 milligrams of calcium per 100 grams while the calcium content of locust bean can reach 300 milligrams per 100 grams.

Besides being the most important source of vegetable protein after that of cereals, legumes can also be an excellent source of calories (300 to 400 calories per 100 grams). Since they can fill protein and caloric deficiencies, they are especially important off-season or in periods of drought when the principal commodity, either cereal or tuber, is lacking.

Excerpted from: *Lozano, Y. "Les légumineuses" ("Plant Protein")* Afrique Agriculture, *no. 50, October 1979, pp. 30-31.*

The Importance of Protein Content in Leaves

If we consult a standard table of nutrient content in vegetables, such as one provided by the Food and Agriculture Organization, we see that the protein content of fresh vegetables hovers around 2 percent.

Systematic analyses of leaves eaten in Senegal and in the Sahel zone were done at ORANA. The higher protein content of some of these leaves was determined. Here are some average protein contents found:

Peanut leaves..5.6%
Amaranthus caudatus................................4.6%
Cassia Tora..6.2%
Jute (*Corchorus olitorius*).........................5.1%
Squash leaves...6.0%
Ficus leaves..6.1%
Cassava leaves..8.3%
Neverdia leaves (*Moringa pterygosperma*)......8.3%
Cow-pea leaves (*Vigna unguiculata*)..............5.3%

The protein of these leaves is generally low in methionine; thus, they are a good supplement to grains that are low in lysine. Furthermore, when the leaves are eaten as shoots, they are usually richer in essential amino acids and more easily digested than mature leaves.

Excerpted from: *Toury, J.* Les légumes et les fruits (Vegetables and Fruits) *ORANA, Dakar, Document A 21, ronéotypé.*

Use of Vegetable Protein for Breast-Fed Infants

It is clear that vegetable protein can easily be used to feed breast-fed infants. To illustrate the possibility of normal growth by relying solely on vegetable protein, we will cite two examples. One case concerns nursing infants, whose growth is affected as soon as any necessary element is lacking. The other case deals with children afflicted with kwashiorkor, which requires a higher than normal intake of necessary amino acids for recovery.

The first example is the result of work begun in Paris in 1930. It involved the search for a replacement product for nursing children who could not tolerate any food of animal origin (complete intolerance to milk products). Two mixtures were fully capable of assuring normal growth in the nursing child: one was made up of 70 percent cream of rice and 30 percent sunflower meal (the oil and hull of the sunflower seeds were removed) and the other, 70 percent cream of rice and 30 percent soy flour. Some vitamins were added, as were malt extracts to ease digestion. In some cases, a bit of powdered milk in small doses (1 to 2 percent of the daily allowance) had to be added to stabilize the weight curve. This formula can be used for several months with excellent results (cf. Thesis of Willemin-Cloq: "Use of Vegetable Protein in the Infant Diet," Paris, 1930). Here we see the grain-legume association adapted to children's diets: grain-oil seed (rice-sunflower) and grain-legume (rice-soy).

The other example is, perhaps, more demonstrative, for it concerns children stricken with kwashiorkor who need great quantities of high-quality protein. This work was done in India where kwashiorkor is prevalent and where animal products are not readily available. One hundred thirty-four children afflicted with the disease were treated. Some received the classic treatment with powdered skim milk; others were treated with only the most common vegetable products: rice and chick-peas. The following preparation made the chick-peas easily digestible for sick children: first, the chick-peas were soaked, allowing germination to begin over a 40-hour period. They were next dried in the sun and the oven, hulled, and ground into a fine meal. Additional vitamins were added in the form of fresh fruit. The recovery of children fed with chick-peas and rice was slightly longer than those fed with powdered milk, but the results were nonetheless satisfactory and the children recovered completely (Venkatachalam et al., 1956).

As a doctor in the South of Morocco, I had to treat nutritional edemas in a population too poor to eat animal products regularly. I was able to balance the diet and cure the edema with the most common food products available in the area—barley, lentils, and almonds—without the help of powdered milk or other animal products that these sick children would never be able to consume on a regular basis. These cases of edema were primarily caused by either poor food associations or by cooking methods that left the food too coarse to be properly digested. This is often the case when children are put on an adult diet directly after weaning because the food is usually under cooked and overspiced.

Excerpted from: *Parodi, P. "Efficacité des moyens pauvres dans l'aide au Tiers-Monde" ("Effectiveness of Poor Means in Aid to the Third World") L'Arche, Ceilhes (Hérault-France), 1971, p. 36.*

Spirulina, Protein Source

Spirulina, an alga found in the desert of Chad, has been used to feed mankind for many centuries. It contains 70 percent high-quality protein (70 percent of its dry weight), and it opens vast horizons for tropical and semitropical countries suffering from malnutrition.

Experiments performed to produce this alga at a low cost and in the simplest way possible were very interesting. It was found that the protein necessary for an entire village could be produced by the people themselves, thus eliminating industrial, administrative, sales, and transportation costs, while providing a small profit to aid the needy.

Fox (1973) shows us how to prepare *Spirulina* in a basin and describes a successful experiment in India that was financed by the Association to Combat Malnutrition with Simplified Alga-Crops (ALMA).

Spirulina needs exposure to sunlight that is not too intense. The water in which it is grown should be at room temperature, and the water level in the basin must be constant. The materials for a small village system cost about 1,200 francs, an amount that can be paid off in four years. It is quite interesting to compare the nutritive value of *Spirulina* with that of an egg (see table 9–1).

Table 9-1   Essential amino acid content of Spirulina and the egg

Amino acids	*S. platensis*	Egg
Arginine	7.8	6.1
Cystine	0.7	2.3
Histidine	1.8	2.4
Isoleucine	6.4	5.6
Leucine	10.4	8.8
Lysine	4.4	6.8
Methionine	2.2	3.5
Phenylalanine	5.4	6.0
Threonine	5.4	5.1
Tryptophan	0.8	1.4
Tyrosine	5.0	4.3
Valine	7.5	6.7

Source: "Spirulina platensis, Geitler et Spirulina Geitleri" de J. de Toni, 1971, Marseille, par le pharmacien F. Busson.

Excerpted from: *Fox, R. "Un bassin expérimental pour la culture de la* Spiruline" *("An Experimental Basin for* Spirulina *Culture") Navsari I, May 1973 (summary of the article by A. Marecaux, GRET, 1980).*

Question 10

Do vitamin deficiencies exist? Can vitamins be manufactured for free?

Vitamin deficiencies occur frequently in both developed and developing countries. They result in increased susceptibility to disease and in severe cases are the direct cause of disease (Delaunay, 1964).

In industrialized countries, in spite of a varied and abundant food supply, vitamin deficiencies are not rare. In Louisiana, 45 percent of children less than six years old suffer from a vitamin A deficiency. The same deficiency occurs in 60 percent of all children and adolescents in Texas and in 45 percent of all Canadian women from 20 to 38 years of age ("Nutrition Canada," 1973).

Such deficiencies can be easily explained: increasing amounts of food are refined, canned, or have traveled a long way from their source, losing a good deal of their original vitamin content.

In developing countries the same phenomenon is made worse by the fact that the diet is less varied. Vitamin deficiencies are almost always more serious in cities than in rural areas where unrefined food is more common and where vegetables and fruits are almost always eaten immediately after picking.

Thus, in Senegal, according to a 1980 study, the percent of the minimum daily requirement consumed in rural zones was 205 percent for vitamin A, 130 percent for vitamin B_1, and 55 percent for vitamin B_2. The calorie and protein intakes in Dakar were higher than in the rural areas, but vitamin A

145

intake was only 81 percent with consumption of vitamins B_1 and B_2 being only 77 and 39 percent, respectively.

Several simple precautions can prevent the destruction of vitamin content in food:

- eat unrefined food;
- pick fruits and vegetables when ripe;
- eat vegetables shortly after picking them (in temperate climates, leafy vegetables can lose up to 90 percent of their vitamin C in several days when stored at room temperature; in tropical climates, vitamin loss is even more rapid);
- limit the consumption of canned goods;
- avoid cooking vegetables too long in a lot of water to prevent leaching of water-soluble vitamins.

Everyone can "manufacture" vitamins at home for free by using two remarkable processes: sprouting and fermentation. A sprouting seed is the most nearly perfect, least expensive vitamin "factory" (see table 10-1). In three days of sprouting, the amount of vitamin C in soybeans goes from 0 to 72 milligrams per 100 grams. The amount of carotene (a precursor of vitamin A) contained in sprouting grains and legumes is multiplied two to four times in the same amount of time (see chart 7). The amounts of vitamins B_2 (riboflavin) and B_{12} also increase in considerable proportions (see tables 10-2 and 10-3). These observations confirm the benefits of traditional sprouted food, such as soy sprouts or bulgur. Lactic acid fermentation is also accompanied by vitamin synthesis, notably vitamin C and the B vitamins (see question 7). Van Veen et al. (1968) found that fermented rice, a food frequently consumed in Ecuador, contained about two times more riboflavin than nonfermented rice. Also, the riboflavin content of rice flour after fermentation by *Bacillus subtilis* was four times greater than that of nonfermented flour.

Table 10-1	Nutritive content of wheat, wheat sprouts, alfalfa sprouts, and soy sprouts (mg/100 g)			
	Wheat	Wheat sprouts (dehydrated)	Alfalfa sprouts (dehydrated)	Fresh soy sprouts*
Protein (%)	12.10	25.20	20.00	6.00
Calcium	41.00	90.00	1,750.00	50.00
Phosphorus	372.00	1,100.00	250.00	65.00
Magnesium	120.00	400.00	310.00	—
Iron	3.30	8.00	35.00	1.20
Copper	0.17	1.30	2.00	—
Vitamin A	0.12	—	13.20	—
Vitamin B_1	0.55	1.00	0.80	0.23
Vitamin B_2	0.12	2.50	1.80	0.20
Vitamin B_3	4.30	5.00	5.00	0.80
Vitamin C	0.00	1.00	176.00	10.00

*The nutritive content given here for soy sprouts is much lower than wheat and alfalfa sprouts as the soy was freshly sprouted, containing 86% water, while the wheat and alfalfa sprouts were dried and contained 10 to 12% water.

Excerpted from: Aubert, C. *Une autre assiette* Éd. Debard, Paris, 1979, p. 300.

Table 10-2   Vitamin content of seeds before and after 5 days of sprouting (mg/kg)

	Vitamin B₂ (riboflavin)		Vitamin B₃ (niacin)		Vitamin B₁ (thiamine)		Vitamin H (biotin)	
	Not sprouted	Sprouted	Not sprouted	Sprouted	Not sprouted	Sprouted	Not sprouted	Sprouted
Barley	1.3	8.3	72	129	—	7.9	0.4	1.2
Corn	1.2	3.0	17	40	6.2	5.5	0.3	0.7
Hay	0.6	12.4	11	48	10.0	11.5	1.2	1.8
Soy	2.0	9.1	27	49	10.7	9.6	1.1	3.5
Lima beans	0.9	4.0	11	41	4.5	6.2	0.1	0.4
Mung beans	1.2	10.0	26	70	8.8	10.3	0.2	1.0
Peas	0.7	7.3	31	32	7.2	9.2	—	0.5

Tables 10-2, 10-3, and 10-4 excerpted from: Kulvinskas, V. "Sprout for the Love of Everybody," Omangod Press, 21st Century Publication PUF, P.O. Box 702, Fairfield, IA 52556, 1978.

Table 10-3   Vitamin B_{12} content of cereals and legumes in sprouting process (mg/kg)

	Before sprouting	After sprouting 2 days	After sprouting 4 days
Mung beans	0.61	0.81	1.53
Lentils	0.43	0.42	2.37
Peas	0.36	1.27	2.36

Chart 7

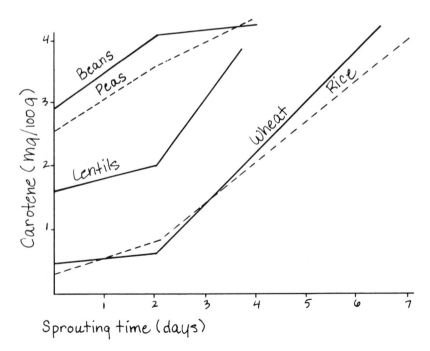

Table 10-4   Vitamin C content of legume seeds in sprouting process

Sprouting time	Vitamin C
Not yet sprouted	Traces
24 hours after sprouting	7 to 8 mg/100 g
48 hours after sprouting	10 to 12 mg/100 g
72 hours after sprouting	12 to 14 mg/100 g

Table 10-5   Protein and vitamin content in soy flour and fermented soy products

	Soy flour	Dried natto (fermented product)	Dried miso (fermented product)
Protein (%)	31.19	31.71	24.3
Vitamin B_1 (μg/g)	0.3	1.0	0.6
Vitamin B_2 (μg/g)	3.0	8.6	1.95
Vitamin B_{12} (μg/g)	0.033	0.16	0.07

Excerpted from: National Academy of Sciences, "Meeting Protein Needs of Infants and Preschool Children," National Research Council, Washington, D.C., 1961, Pub. 843.

Supplementary Readings for Question 10

> Do vitamin deficiencies exist? Can vitamins be manufactured for free?

Nutritional Deficiencies and Resistance to Infection

One of the most notable effects of nutritional deficiencies is the impact they have on an organism's resistance to infections. In most cases, nutritional deficiencies lower resistance of the host to bacteria, rickettsia, and helminthiasis (parasitic intestinal worms). They can increase or lower resistance to protozoa and generally increase resistance to viruses.

The pro-infectious action, lowering host resistance, is due mainly to an attack on the body's defense mechanisms, primarily those that form antibodies. The anti-infectious action paradoxically associated with the same deficiency is caused by the lack of a vital metabolite, making reproduction and survival impossible for the parasite or virus.

General studies of vitamin deficiencies have revealed that a vitamin A deficiency promotes infection, while a vitamin B deficiency can either promote or fight infection, depending on the specific case.

Excerpted from: Delaunay, A. *"Carences nutritionnelles et résistance aux infections"* (*"A Nutritional Deficiency and Resistance to Infections"*) Annales de la Nutrition et de l'Alimentation, Éd. CNRS, vol. 18, no. 2, 1964, pp. 1-41.

Question 11

Can health be improved by changes in the diet?

A country's state of health depends, in large measure, on what it eats. In industrialized countries, numerous diseases are caused by overindulgent, imbalanced diets. Heart disease, many types of cancer, and diabetes are directly related to eating habits: excessive consumption of animal fats and sugar, insufficient fiber, general overeating, chemical pollutants in food.

In developing countries, the main problem is, of course, malnutrition. But, as a general rule, this is due more to class structure than to agricultural capability. In urban areas, the poor may not have the money to buy themselves food and do not have the land on which to grow their own. This situation is aggravated when native cuisine (unrefined grains, legumes, high-protein vegetables, nuts and seeds), rich in nutrients, is abandoned for food that is often deficient in protein, vitamins, and minerals (see table 11–1).

Unlike the inhabitants of industrialized countries, people in urban areas of poor countries do not have easy access to fresh meat, dairy products, fruits, or vegetables to compensate for the nutritional deficiencies of refined food. Therefore, as food production methods are developed in Third World countries, it is important to avoid making some of the same errors that have been made in industrialized countries.

Let's take another look at the most widespread mistakes and the most serious consequences:

● The replacement of breast feeding with formulas;
● The gradual replacement of grains with tubers (This change was noted in nineteenth-century Europe with the potato and

153

Table 11-1	Percentage of recommended amounts of dietary nutrients consumed in Senegal (Dakar and rural zones)	
	Dakar	Rural zones*
Calories	96	88
Protein	154	140
Calcium	42	103
Iron	83	207
Vitamin A	81	205
Vitamin B_1	77	140
Vitamin B_2	39	55
Vitamin PP	176	207
Vitamin C	223	248

*Regional averages for Diourbel, Casamance, and Kedougou.
These figures show that although inhabitants of Dakar have a richer diet (more calories and more protein) than those of rural zones, the recommended allowances for minerals and vitamins, expressed in percentages, are much lower. This is due to the large role played by foods that have many calories and few nutrients, such as sugar, refined grains, and fats.

Excerpted from: CRDI "État nutritionnel de la population du Sahel" Ottawa, 1980.

is quite noticeable in certain African countries where cassava is eaten in increasing quantities. Since tubers are much less rich in protein than grains, protein deficiencies are quick to appear, unless consumption of meat, fish, dairy products, or legumes is also increased.);

• The use of refined grains in place of whole grains (In Dakar, traditional grains—millet, sorghum, rice—represent only 10 percent of grain consumption; in Asia, white rice has almost completely supplanted brown rice.);

• The consumption of increasing quantities of white sugar (see question 7) (In Africa, white sugar is sold even in the most isolated villages; in Latin America and India, it is gradually replacing much more nutrient-rich unrefined sugar.);

- The increasing consumption of Western foods and drink (refined sugar, canned goods, white flour, beer, cola beverages);
- The lowered consumption of legumes, a good protein source that is potentially available to all levels of the population.

A real health policy must be based on prevention. Caring for the sick is urgent and necessary, but preventing the healthy from becoming sick is just as urgent and necessary and much less costly.

Among the many factors that determine an individual's state of health, food is the one most easily changed. To influence eating habits and improve health, measures must be taken at the agricultural production level, within the food-processing industry, and among the people.

At the agricultural production level, priority should be given to domestic food crops. Use of pesticides and excessive amounts of nitrate fertilizers should be avoided. Development of crops, such as grains, legumes, vegetables, nuts and seeds, and seaweed, that provide food particularly rich in nutrients should be encouraged.

Within the food-processing industry, limitations should be set on the production of overrefined foods and foods that are imbalanced or low in nutrients, such as refined grains, white sugar, canned goods, and artificial drinks. At the same time, alternative technologies which preserve or improve the nutritive value of food (whole-grain-based foods, raw sugar, preservation by drying or fermentation) could be developed.

Other measures that would greatly improve the nutritional status of Third World populations as well as save a great deal of money are:

- encouraging women to breast-feed;
- teaching the basics of a healthy diet;
- making the advantages of local products over imported products known;
- combating the multinational firms' prevalent, often misleading advertising.

Supplementary Readings for Question 11

> Can health be improved by changes in the diet?

Rarity of Deficiencies in "Primitive" Populations

On the African continent, in the Far East, and in other less industrialized regions, you can still find grains with vitamin and mineral contents many times higher than the grains consumed by the earth's peoples as a whole.

This explains, up to a certain point, the rarity of nutritional deficiencies in populations that remain isolated or almost isolated from civilization. Although these population groups may not have sufficient quantities of food, their diet generally includes local products which are extremely rich in vitamins and minerals.

As we have already seen (question 8), as soon as outside contact is established, traditional diets are forgotten. Bigwood and Trolli (1937) observed this fact in the Belgian Congo where the native diet, based on millet, sorghum, cassava, sweet potato, and some lesser-known foods, maintained the health and fitness of the local population. But as soon as they came to work in factories and adopted a European-type diet, they fell prey to various vitamin and mineral deficiencies—beriberi, pellagra—which quickly decimated them.

Excerpted from: *Castro, J. de* Géopolitique de la faim (Geo-Politics of Hunger) *Éditions Ouvrières, Paris, 1952.*

The Rise of Modern Diseases
in the Third World

Diabetes is an almost universal sickness. It spares no continent, even though the rates of its prevalence are extremely variable from one country to another. In Africa, this disease's progression has drawn a great deal of attention. From 1960 to 1970 the ratio of diabetics went from 1 to 4 for every 100 persons hospitalized. In 1965, a diabetes center had to be created in Dakar; it is currently treating over 3,000 patients.

Diabetes is most prevalent among city dwellers. In the capital of Senegal, the rate of prevalence is estimated at 2 percent of the inhabitants and glycosuria after meals has been observed in 1.7 percent. By contrast, the incidence of this sugar-related disease is much lower in the rural areas (Sankale et al., 1974).

Like diabetes, atherosclerosis is also on the rise in developing countries. Myocardial infarctions and arterial conditions in the limbs, formerly unknown in Africans, are becoming more and more common. Such trends definitely constitute a threat for the future.

Excerpted from: *Sankale, M.; Satge, P.; Toury, J.; and Vuylsteke, S.* *"Alimentation et pathologie nutritionnelle en Afrique Noire"* *("Food and Nutritional Pathology in Black Africa") Éd. Maloine, Paris, 1974.*

Conclusion

Throughout the history of the world, agriculture had been man's chief productive activity until the eighteenth century. Then, Western civilization gave priority to the development of industry and wanted to industrialize everything, including agriculture. Therefore, agricultural production has increased considerably in some countries, most often to the detriment of food quality. At the same time, the imbalance between the underfed and the overfed has gone beyond tolerable limits, even though rich countries tolerate the situation very well!

Malnutrition is getting worse in the Third World, while diseases caused by a diet that is unbalanced and too rich are increasing in industrialized countries. If we persist in the present direction, all people might soon find themselves deprived of their most prized possession: health. Health comes before everything—it is necessary for both happiness and a sound development. Promoting the production, distribution, and consumption of food that will preserve man's health is, therefore, a priority for all countries.

Références Bibliographiques

1 Agarwal (A.) "Pesticide Poisoning—Another Third World Disease" *New Scientist*, London, 21-28 December 1978, p. 917.

2 Almeida (S. G. de) "Pérou: La subordination d'une agriculture régionale" *Le Monde Diplomatique*, no. 294, septembre 1978, pp. 7-8.

3 Amin (Collectif sous la direction de S.) "L'agriculture africaine et le capitalisme" Éd. Anthropos—IDEP, Paris, 1975, p. 377.

4 ARES (Application de Recherches sur l'Energie et la Société) "Innovations rurales aux États-Unis" CIIS (Centre d'Information sur les Innovations Sociales), 1979.

5 Armijo (R.) & Coulson (A.) "Épidémiologie du cancer de l'estomac au Chili: le rôle des engrais azotés" *International Journal of Epidemiology*, vol. 4, no. 4, 1975, p. 1.

6 AIT (Asian Institute of Technology—Bangkok) "Séchoir solaire pour le riz" *Afrique Agriculture*, no. 50, octobre 1979, p. 43.

7 Assion (L. G.) "Préservation des stocks de niébé sans résidus: l'huilage des grains" CIT—AUPELF—Université de Yaoundé (Cameroun), 10-12 mai 1979, p. 1.

8 ACTA & CoLuMa (Comité de Lutte contre les Mauvaises Herbes) "Les herbicides et le sol" Paris, 1977, p. 143.

9 Atangana (S.) & all. "Les incidences des barrages sur la santé publique au Cameroun" Document du Ministère de la Santé de la République Unie du Cameroun, Yaoundé, 1978, p. 17.

10 Aubart (C.) "La posidonie: ressource inexploitée" Résumé d'article réalisé par A. Marecaux, GRET, 1980, p. 1.

11 Aubert (C.) *L'agriculture biologique—Pourquoi et comment la pratiquer* Éd. Le Courrier du Livre, Paris, 1977, p. 363.

12 Aubert (C.) *Les aliments fermentés traditionnels, une richesse méconnue* Éd. Terre Vivante, Paris, 1985.

13 Aubert (C.) *L'assiette aux céréales* Éd. Terre Vivante, Paris, 1983.

14 Aubert (C.) "Le lait maternel" *Nature et Progrès*, octobre-novembre-décembre 1974, pp. 21-29.

15 Aubert (C.) "Quelle politique agro-alimentaire pour le Tiers-Monde?" *Nature et Progrès*, no. 76, Paris, septembre-octobre 1982.

16 Aubert (C.) *Une autre assiette* Éd. Debard, Paris, 1979, p. 300.

17 Aykroyd (W. R.) & Doughty (J.) "Le blé dans l'alimentation humaine" FAO, Rome, 1970.

18 Aykroyd (W. R.) & Doughty (J.) "Legumes in Human Nutrition" FAO, Washington, D.C., 1974.

19 Babile (R.) "Additifs alimentaires et anomalies chromosomiques—Étude in vitro" Thèse de Docteur Ingénieur, Institut National Polytechnique de Toulouse, 1978.

20 Basse (M. T.) interview "Nous cherchons à rendre les produits locaux aussi attrayants que les produits importés" *Cérès*, no. 63, juin-juillet 1978, pp. 38-41.

21 Batsch (C.) "Les mésaventures d'une entreprise de maraîchage au Sénégal" *Le Monde Diplomatique*, no. 318, septembre 1980, p. 10.

22 Beguin (Dr. M. H.) "Aliments naturels, dents saines" Éd. de l'Étoile, La Chaux de Fonds, 1979.

23 Bel (F.); Le Pape (Y.); & Mollard (A.) "Analyse énergétique de la production agricole" INRA—IREP, Grenoble, juillet 1978, p. 163.

24 Belloncle (C.) "A l'écoute du paysan" *Cérès*, juin-juillet 1973.

25 Ben Ali (C.) "Politique alimentaire et nutritionnelle en Tunisie" in "La Méditerranée face à la crise alimentaire—Des choix urgents," supplément à la *Lettre d'Information d'Échanges Méditerranée*, no. 24, juin 1980, pp. 78-82.

26 Benoit-Cattin (M.) "Les céréales traditionnelles" *Afrique Agriculture*, no. 50, octobre 1979, p. 29.

27 Bergeret (A.) "Vers une plus large autonomie alimentaire du Tiers-Monde" Thèse de Doctorat, Université de Paris I, juin 1977.

28 Bergeret (A.) & Thery (D.) "Il n'y a pas de mauvaises herbes" *Cérès*, no. 50, mars-avril 1976, pp. 29-32.

29 Bergeret (A.) & all. "Nourrir en harmonie avec l'environnement—Trois études de cas" Éd. Mouton, Paris/La Haye, 1977, p. 298.

30 Berlan (J. P.) "Quelques aspects de la production de semences dans le monde" Entretien in "La Méditerranée face à la crise alimentaire—Des choix urgents," supplément à la *Lettre d'Information d'Échanges Méditerranée*, no. 24, juin 1980, pp. 83-88.

31 Berlan (J. P.) & Rouiller (L.) "Semences—Nouvelles variétés" Entretien in "La Méditerranée face à la crise alimentaire—Des choix urgents," supplément à la *Lettre d'Information d'Échanges Méditerranée*, no. 24, juin 1980, pp. 47-50.

32 Bessis (S.) "L'arme alimentaire" Éd. Maspéro, Paris, 1979.

33 Billaz (R.) "Le mandarinat de la recherche" *Cérès*, janvier-février 1974.

34 Billaz (R.) "Questions à la recherche agronomique tropicale" *Actuel Développement*, no. 4, novembre-décembre 1974.

35 Bircher (R.) "Les Hounza," un peuple qui ignore la maladie Éd. V. Attinger, Neuchâtel, 1962.

36 Blanchemain (A.) "A propos d'aménagement des parcours forestiers: Quelle responsabilité?" *Forêt Méditerranéenne*, tome II, no. 1, juillet 1980, pp. 61-66.

37 Bolton (M.) "Élevage du crocodile en Papouasie—Nouvelle Guinée" *Revue Mondiale de Zootechnie* Éd. FAO, no. 34, 1980, pp. 15-22.

38 Botazzi (M.) "Contre la faim, un autre développement" *Croissance des Jeunes Nations*, no. 215, mars 1980, pp. 33-35.

39 Bougeois (D.) "Pesticides: le 2,4,5-T" *Nature et Progrès*, no. 49, janvier-février-mars 1976, p. 23.

40 Brammer (H.) "Il y a des innovations qui se passent d'experts" *Cérès*, mars-avril 1980, pp. 24-28. Cet article a été aussi publié sous le titre "Paysans du Bangladesh" dans *Les Quatre Saisons du Jardinage*, no. 5, novembre-décembre 1980, pp. 80-88.

41 Bull (D.) "A Growing Problem—Pesticides and the Third World Poor" OXFAM, Oxford, 1982.

42 BIT (Bureau International du Travail) "Technologies appropriées dans les industries de transformation alimentaire et de conservation des fruits dans quatre pays de la CEAO: Haute-Volta, Mali, Niger, Sénégal" Addis-Ababa, 1982.

43 Castel (P.) "Agro-business: le racket de la faim" *Croissance des Jeunes Nations*, no. 195, mai 1978, pp. 19-26.

44 Castro (J. de) "Géographie de la faim" Éd. du Seuil, Collection Point Politique no. 52, Paris, 1972, p. 350.

45 Castro (J. de) *Géopolitique de la faim* Éditions Ouvrières, Paris, 1952.

46 Chaboussou (F.) "Fumures, traitements et autres facteurs extrinsèques conditionnent la résistance de la plante" *Encyclopédie permanente d'agriculture biologique*, Éd. Debard, Paris 1, Phytopathologie, Fumures, pp. 1-14, 1974.

47 Chaboussou (F.) "Les plantes malades des pesticides" Éd. Debard, Paris, 1980.

48 Cheret (I.) "L'eau" Éd. du Seuil, Collection "Société" no. 20, Paris, 1967, p. 128.

49 Chonchol (J.) "L'échec des solutions productivistes" *Politique Aujourd'hui*, no. 1-2, janvier-février 1980, pp. 61-70.

50 Chonchol (J.) "Espaces ruraux et planification du développement" *Le Monde Diplomatique*, no. 304, juillet 1979, pp. 12-14.

51 Colas (R.) "La pollution des eaux" Presses Universitaires de France, Collection "Que sais-je?" no. 983, Paris, 1962, p. 128.

52 Collombon (J. M.) "Demain une agriculture plus écologique—Prémisses et promesses" Polycopié, juin 1980, p. 16.

53 Collombon (J. M.) "Les jardins de marécage de Xochimilco au Mexique" *Les Quatre Saisons du Jardinage*, no. 3, juillet-août 1980, pp. 77-83.

54 Collombon (J. M.) "Production vivrière traditionnelle en Ethiopie" *Les Quatre Saisons du Jardinage*, no. 2, mai-juin 1980, pp. 65-70.

55 Collombon (J. M.) "Les techniques agricoles des Indiens Miskitos d'Amérique Centrale" *Les Quatre Saisons du Jardinage*, no. 1, mars-avril 1980, pp. 69-74.

56 Collombon (J. M.) "Technologies appropriées pour une stratégie alternative de développement" CCPD—Documents (Conseil Oecuménique des Églises) no. 16, juin 1979.

57 Comité d'Information Sahel "Qui se nourrit de la famine en Afrique?" Petite Collection Maspéro, no. 153, Paris, 1975, p. 200.

58 Comte (M. C.) "Alimentation infantile: les dangers du biberon" *Cérès*, mai-juin 1978, no. 63, pp. 8-9.

59 Conti (L.) "Qu'est ce que l'écologie?" Petite Collection Maspéro, no. 300, Paris, 1978, p. 157. Original title: "Che cos'è l'ecologia" Gabriele Mazzotta, Milan.

60 Cottingham (J.) "Le biberon qui tue" Service Féminin International d'Information, Carouge (Suisse), 1976, p. 3.

61 Couet (J. F.) & Bremond (J.) "Pays sous-développés ou pays en voie de développement?" Hatier, Paris, 1978.

62 CRDI "État nutritionnel de la population du Sahel," Ottawa, 1980.

63 Curie (M.) "Pollution autour d'une sucrerie—De l'eau noire et nauséabonde dans le canal de la Somme" *Le Monde*, no. 8 343, octobre-novembre 1971, p. 10.

64 Custot (F.) "Inflation et qualité" *Coopération, Distribution, Consommation,* septembre 1975. Cet article est également paru dans *Problèmes Économiques,* no. 1 440, 10 janvier 1975.

65 Dajoz (R.) "Les insecticides" Presses Universitaires de France, Collection "Que sais-je?" no. 829, Paris, 1969, p. 128.

66 Dalleine (E.) "En Bretagne, baisse des rendements et fatigue des sols" *Agri-Sept,* no. 778, 11 mai 1980, p. 23.

67 Debry (G.) "L'athérosclérose, maladie des trop nourris" *Science et Vie,* Hors Série no. 130 ("L'homme et son alimentation"), pp. 72-80.

68 Degremont (Sté) "Mémento technique de l'eau" Rueil-Malmaison, 1972, p. 100.

69 Delaunay (A.) "Carences nutritionnelles et résistance aux infections" *Annales de la Nutrition et de l'Alimentation* Éd. CNRS, vol. 18, no. 2, 1964, pp. 1-41.

70 Delwaulle (J. C.) "Désertification de l'Afrique au Sud du Sahara" *Bois et Forêts des Tropiques,* no. 149, mai-juin 1973.

71 Dorange (J. L.) "Effets mutagènes des nitrates et des nitrites" *Annales de la Nutrition et de l'Alimentation* Éd. CNRS, vol. 30, no. 5-6, 1976.

72 Dorozynski (A.) "Mercure; des taux alarmants dans les poissons de la Méditerranée" *Sciences et Vie,* no. 687, décembre 1974, pp. 52-53.

73 Drucker (L. B.) "On the Island of Luzon, the Igorot Culture and Rice Terraces Developed Together" *Sierra Club Bulletin,* Albany (Canada), vol. 63, no. 8, October-November-December 1978, pp. 22-26. Extraits parus en français in *Problèmes Politiques et Sociaux,* no. 363, 25 mai 1979, pp. 16-17.

74 Dumont (R.) "L'agriculture voltaïque dans le piège de la dépendance" *Le Monde Diplomatique,* mars 1978, pp. 1-22.

75 Dumont (R.) "La croissance . . . de la famine" Éd. du Seuil, Paris, 1975.

76 Dumont (R.) *False Start in Africa*, André Deutsch, London, 1968, pp. 58-59.

77 Dumont (R.) "Réforme agraire; par où commencer?" *Cérès*, no. 70, juillet-août 1979, pp. 37-40.

78 Dumont (R.) "Terres vivantes" Éd. Plon, Collection "Terre Humaine," Paris, 1961, p. 334.

79 Dumont (R.) "L'Utopie ou la Mort" Éd. du Seuil, Collection Point Politique no. 67, Paris, 1974, p. 190.

80 Dumont (R.) & Mottin (M. F.) "L'Afrique étranglée" Éd. du Seuil, Paris, 1980, p. 265.

81 Dupin (H.) "Le modèle alimentaire occidental" *Jeune Afrique*, Dossier Bis "La crise alimentaire mondiale" janvier-juin 1975, pp. 58-60.

82 Dupin (H.) & Brun (T.) "Évolution de l'alimentation dans les pays en voie de développement" *D'aceveloppement et Santé*, no. 11, p. 11.

83 Échanges Méditerranée "La Méditerranée face à la crise alimentaire—Des choix urgents" Dossier de synthèse du Colloque d'Arles, 24-26 avril 1980, Supplément à la *Lettre d'Information d'Échanges Méditerranée*, no. 24, juin 1980, p. 130.

84 Eckolm (E. P.) "La schistosomiase, une maladie des pauvres . . . et du développement" *Cérès*, janvier-février 1978, pp. 37-41.

85 Eckolm (E. P.) "La terre sans arbres" Éd. R. Laffont, 1977, p. 330.

86 ENSAM—IFARC (École Nationale Supérieure Agronomique de Montpellier—Institut pour la Formation Agricole et Rurale en Régions Chaudes) "Production de boissons fermentées artisanales au Shaba (Zaïre)" Fichier Documentaire "Agronomie des Régions Chaudes" (FICHARC), fasc. 1.

87 Egg (J.) "Un effet de la rente pétrolière au Nigeria" *Le Monde Diplomatique*, no. 314, mai 1980, p. 17.

88 Egger (Dr. K. E.) "Vers l'agroécologie optimale—Étude de la conservation des sols dans quelques ORD en Haute Volta" Polycopié—Ouagadougou/Heidelberg, février 1980, p. 60.

89 Egger (Dr. K.) & Zeuner (Dr. T. H.) "Une conception écologique pour l'agriculture" Rapport délivré à SEM le Ministre de l'Agriculture et de l'Élevage de la République Rwandaise, juin 1976, p. 28.

90 Eide (A.) "Cultiver de tout partout" *Cérès*, no. 43.

91 El Husseini (A.) "Un fourrage au rendement éléphantesque" *Le CRDI explore*, vol. 9, no. 3, octobre 1980.

92 Escoffier-Lambiotte (Dr.) "Régimes alimentaires et maladies de civilisation" *Le Monde*, no. 9 534, 17 septembre 1975, p. 17.

93 Etoundi (O.) "Quatre complexes de grande envergure sur les rails" *Cameroun Tribune*, no. 1 059, 31 décembre 1977, p. 5.

94 Euseby (C.) "La bilharziose et le sous-développement: pour une approche globale du problème" *Tiers-Monde*, tome XX, no. 80, octobre-décembre 1979, pp. 773-94.

95 Faivre (J.) & all. "Les méthémoglobinémies induites par l'ingestion de nitrites et de nitrates" *Annales de la Nutrition et de l'Alimentation* Éd. CNRS, vol. 30, no. 5-6, 1976.

96 Fauconnier (D.) "Le soja pour mieux nourrir l'Quest Africain" *Afrique Agriculture*, no. 59, juillet 1980, pp. 12-13.

97 Favier (J. C.) "Influence des techniques traditionnelles de préparation du manioc et du sorgho" CIT—AUPELF—Université de Yaoundé (Cameroun), 5-10 décembre 1979, p. 1.

98 Faye (J.); Gallali (T.); & Billaz (R.) "L'agronomie vécue: un défi pour les modèles planifiés?" *Environnement Africain*, vol. II, 4 & III, 1, novembre 1977, pp. 39-48.

99 Feder (E.) "Le loup déguisé en brebis" *Cérès*, no. 52, juillet-août 1976, pp. 40-44.

100 Fevrier (R.) Entretien in "La Méditerranée face à la crise alimentaire—Des choix urgents," supplément à la *Lettre d'Information d'Échanges Méditerranée*, no. 24, juin 1980, pp. 21-23.

101 Fevrier (R.) interview—*Entreprises agricoles*, no. 98, janvier 1978, Dossier "La production agricole dans l'impasse?" pp. 31-38.

102 Fevrier (R.) & Poly (J.) "Évolution prévisible du monde rural et du secteur agro-alimentaire" Note pour la 4th Conférence de Travail des Directeurs de la Recherche Agronomique, OCDE, Paris, novembre 1979.

103 Fleury (A.) & Mollard (A.) "Agriculture, système social et environnement" IREP—CNEEJA, Grenoble, juillet 1976, p. 327.

104 Fondation Simon I. Patino et Pro Bolivia Projet Agrobiologique Cochabamba, Bolivia, PAC, 1981.

105 FAO (Food and Agriculture Organization) "L'emploi des Matières Organiques comme engrais" Rapport d'une Consultation d'Experts à Rome, 2-6 décembre 1974, Bulletin Pédagogique de la FAO, no. 25, Rome, 1975.

106 Fox (R.) "Un bassin expérimental pour la culture de la *Spiruline*" Navsari I, mai 1973 (résumé d'article par A. Marecaux, GRET, 1980).

107 Franz (Dr. J. M.) "Coccinelles contre pucerons: découvrez la lutte biologique" *Les Quatre Saisons du Jardinage*, no. 18, janvier-février 1983, pp. 60-67.

108 Franz (Dr. J. M.) "La protection biologique des végétaux dans l'Empire du Milieu" *Les Quatre Saisons du Jardinage*, no. 18, janvier-février 1983, pp. 53-58.

109 Froc (J.) "La pollution des graisses animales par les pesticides organochlorés" Thèse de Doctorat, Université de Paris XI, 1977.

110 Fyot (R.) "La valorisation industrielle d'une boisson traditionnelle: le vin de palme pasteurisé" *Techniques et Développement*, juillet-août 1973, pp. 28-29.

111 Gariboldi (F.) "The Parboiling Process" FAO, Washington, D.C., 1974, pp. 1-2.

112 Garreau (G.) "L'agrobusiness" Éd. Calmann-Lévy, Paris, 1977, p. 300.

113 Gast (M.) & Sigaut (F.) "Les techniques de conservation des grains à long terme" CNRS, Paris, 1979.

114 George (S.) "Stratégie d'intervention des pays industrialisés dans les systèmes alimentaires des pays périphériques" Thèse de Doctorat de 3d cycle, Paris, 1978.

115 George (S.) "Le Tiers-Monde face à ses riches clients" *Le Monde Diplomatique*, no. 300, mars 1979, pp. 18-20.

116 Girin (M.) "L'élevage des poissons marins" *La Recherche*, no. 107, janvier 1980, pp. 36-44.

117 Giroud (P. & A.) "Régimes insuffisamment vitaminés et microbes de sortie" Compte rendu des Séances de la Société de Biologie, Séance du 18 juin 1938, tome CXXVIII, 1938, p. 606.

118 Gopalan (C.) "Les terribles séquelles de la malnutrition" *Le Courrier de l'UNESCO*, mai 1975.

119 Griffon (D.) "Le séchage—Recherche pour envisager des unités villageoises polyvalentes" *Afrique Agriculture*, no. 50, octobre 1979, pp. 42-43.

120 Grolleaud (M.) "Sahel: le pouvoir des greniers" *Croissance des Jeunes Nations*, no. 215, mars 1980, pp. 16-18.

121 GASCA (Groupe d'Assistance pour le Stockage des Grains en Afrique) "Les pertes: une question de poids, de qualité et d'argent" *Afrique Agriculture*, no. 50, octobre 1979, p. 28.

122 GRET (Groupe de Recherches et d'Échanges Technologiques), Paris. Très nombreuses fiches techniques; quelques titres:
T 152: Le pyrèthre insecticide.
T 176: Séchoir solaire basculant.
T 185: Compostage de matières organiques avec la fosse fumière.
T 196: Fertilisation par roches siliceuses broyées.
T 197: (Nature et progrès.)
T 207: Le piège à rongeurs de Kornaka.
T 215: Les sources d'azote (N. et P.).
T 264: Séchoir solaire à fruits (Brace Research Institute).
T 300: Séchage direct des fruits au soleil (VITA).
T 302: Séchoir solaire avec ventilateur (BRI).
T 308: Choix d'une micro-rizerie moderne.
T 342: Techniques de compostage au Bangladesh.

123 GRET "Cultures associées en milieu tropical" Ministère des relations extérieures, Paris, 1982.

124 Hadaci (M. L.) "Contribution à l'étude de l'intoxication par parathion en Algérie" Thèse de Doctorat, Université d'Alger, Faculté de Médecine et de Pharmacie, 1968.

125 Howard (Sir A.) "Testament agricole: Pour une agriculture naturelle" Vie et Action, Lille, 1970.

126 IRAT (Institut de Recherches Agronomiques Tropicales et des Cultures Vivrières)—Extrait du rapport de synthèse 80—Agronomie, mars 1981. République de Haute-Volta, Ministère de l'Enseignement Supérieur et de la Recherche Scientifique.

127 Kallqvist (T.) & Meadows (B.) "Concentrations d'insecticides dans l'environnement rural kényan" *Environnement Africain*, vol. II, 4 & III, 1, novembre 1977.

128 KATALYSE—UMWELTGRUPPE—Chemie in Lebensmitteln zweitausendeins, Francfort, 1982.

129 King (F. H.) *Farmers of Forty Centuries*, Rodale Press, 1911.

130 Kulvinskas (V.) "Sprout for the Love of Everybody" Omangod Press, 21st Century Publication PUF, P.O. Box 702, Fairfield, IA 52556, 1978.

131 Labonne (M.) "Le déficit céréalier—D'où vient-il? Qui frappera-t-il? Quelle politique adopter?" *Afrique Agriculture*, no. 50, octobre 1979, pp. 24-25.

132 Lancrenon (P.) "Industrie des engrais—Dépendante de ses matières premières, elle s'interroge sur son avenir" *Agri-Sept*, no. 804, 17 octobre 1980, pp. 20-21.

133 Langley (P.) "Technologies pour l'écodéveloppement" *Environnement Africain*, vol. II, 4 & III, 1, novembre 1977.

134 Langley (P.); N'Gom (M.); & David (P.) "Technologies villageoises dans l'Afrique de l'Quest et du Centre" Fabrication du gari, de la farine de mil et de l'huile d'arachide. UNICEF, 1979.

135 Lederer (J.) *Alimentation et Cancer* Éd. Nauwelaerts/ Maloine, Louvain/Paris, 1977.

136 Legarrec (E.) "La grande bataille des oléagineux" *Le Monde Diplomatique*, no. 299, février 1979, pp. 16-17.

137 Lesca (P.) "La Dioxine et le Cancer" *La Recherche*, no. 114, septembre 1980, pp. 977-79.

138 Linblad (C.) & Druben (L.) "Small Farm Grain Storage" Action/Peace Corps, September 1976, p. 12.

139 Lockeretz (W.) et al. "Organic Farming in the Corn Belt" *Science*, vol. 211, 6 February 1981, pp. 540-47.

140 Lowy (R.) & Manchon (P.) "Effets toxiques divers des nitrates et des nitrites" *Annales de la Nutrition et de l'Alimentation* Éd. CNRS, vol. 30, no. 5-6, 1976.

141 Lozano (Y.) "Les légumineuses" *Afrique Agriculture*, no. 50, octobre 1979, pp. 30-31.

142 MacDowell (J.) "Technologies appropriées pour vaincre la malnutrition" *Contact* (Commission Médicale Chrétienne—Conseil Oecuménique des Églises), no. 36, juillet 1978.

143 Mackay (Dr. F.) "Étude analytique et critique de l'oeuvre de W. A. Price (Thèse de doctorat)" *L'Alimentation Normale*, no. 21-22, AFRAN, Paris, 1959.

144 Malick (S.) "Un projet d'allègement du travail des femmes au Mali" Les carnets de l'Enfance, no. 36, "Alléger le travail des femmes" UNICEF, Genève, octobre-décembre 1976, pp. 66-86.

145 Marloie (M.) "L'abondance mal gérée" *Le Monde Diplomatique*, no. 314, mai 1980, p. 14.

146 Marloie (M.) "Des producteurs et des consommateurs façonnés par les échanges internationaux" *Faim et Développement*, Dossier 48 D, août-septembre 1976.

147 Mazoyer (M. L.) "Impasses et perspectives" dans "Le Point Critique" dir. par Morazé (C.), "Sciences et techniques au service du développement agricole," l'IEDES: Collection Tiers-Monde, PUF, 1982. Passage reproduit avec l'autorisation de l'auteur.

148 Meillassoux (C.) "700,000 paysans de la vallée du Sénégal . . ." *Le Monde Diplomatique*, no. 314, mai 1980, p. 15.

149 Mercier (J. R.) "Énergie et Agriculture" Éd. Debard, Paris, 1978, p. 190.

150 Messe (J. L.) "Agriculture biologique dans le Tiers-Monde" *Nature et Progrès*, janvier-février-mars 1978, pp. 4-9.

151 Moore Lappé (F.) *Diet for a Small Planet*, revised edition, Ballantine, New York, 1978, p. 447.

152 Moore Lappé (F.) "Sans viande et sans regrets" Éd. L'Étincelle, Montréal, 1976.

153 Moore Lappé (F.) & Collins (J.) "Les huit mythes de la faim" *Cérès*, no. 58, juillet-août 1977, pp. 24-30.

154 Moore Lappé (F.) & Collins (J.) "L'industrie de la faim" Éd. L'Étincelle, Paris, 1976.

155 Mosse (A.) "Les facteurs de risque nutritionnels en pathologie cardiovasculaire et leur prévention" *Soins*, tome 25, no. 7, 5 avril 1980.

156 Musalem Lopez (O.) "Mexique: une forme de multinationalisation" *Le Monde Diplomatique*, no. 294, septembre 1978, pp. 14-16.

157 Mutsaers (H. J. W.) "Mixed cropping experiments with maize and groundnuts" Communication no. 1, Département de l'Agriculture, ENSA Yaoundé (Cameroun), 1976.

158 Nolle (J.) Documentation Matériel à traction animale: SINE, ARIANA, TROPICULTEUR, K-NOL..., Établissements MOUZON S.A. (Mouy).

159 Nyerere (J. K.) *Freedom and Socialism*, Oxford University Press, Oxford, 1968, pp. 342-43.

160 Oke (O. L.) "La transformation traditionnelle des aliments au Nigeria" *Environnement Africain*, vol. III, 3-4, no. 11-12, 1979.

161 Omo-Fadaka (J.) "Développement: la troisième voie" *Environnement Africain*, vol. II, 4 & III, 1, novembre 1977.

162 OCDE (Organisation de Coopération et de Développement Économique) "Rapport du groupe d'animation sur la lutte contre les ennemis des cultures vivrières des petits agriculteurs dans les pays en développement" OCDE, Paris, mars 1977, p. 72.

163 OMS (Organisation Mondiale de la Santé) "Épidémiologie et Prophylaxie de la Schistosomiase" Rapport d'un Comité d'Experts de l'OMS, no. 372, OMS, Genève, 1967.

164 OMS "Utilisation des virus dans la lutte contre les insectes nuisibles" Rapport d'un Comité d'Experts FAO—OMS (Réunion 22-27 novembre 1972), no. 531, OMS, Genève, 1973.

165 OMS "Écologie des vecteurs et lutte antivectorielle en santé publique" Rapport d'un Comité d'Experts de l'OMS, no. 561, OMS, Genève, 1975.

166 OMS "Risques pour la santé liés aux nouveaux polluants de l'environnement" Rapport d'un Comité d'Experts de l'OMS, no. 586, OMS, Genève, 1976.

167 OMS "Résidus de pesticides dans les produits alimentaires" Rapport d'un Comité d'Experts FAO—OMS, no. 612, OMS, Genève, 1977.

168 Parodi (P.) "Efficacité des moyens pauvres dans l'aide au Tiers-Monde" L'Arche, Ceilhes (Hérault-France), 1971, p. 36.

169 Parodi (P.) "Robustesse et Alimentation" *L'Alimentation Normale* (Édité par l'AFRAN), no. 21-22, 1959.

170 Perelman (M.) "Le modèle est-il si efficace?" *Le Monde Diplomatique*, no. 294, septembre 1978, pp. 6-7.

171 Picot (Dr. H.) "L'aménagement de la vallée du Bandama" *Bulletin de la Société de Pathologie Exotique*, no. 2, mars-avril 1976, pp. 156-62.

172 Pimentel (D. & M.) "Compter les kilocalories" *Cérès*, no. 59, septembre-octobre 1977, pp. 17-20.

173 Poleman (T. T.) "A double tranchant" *Cérès*, no. 60, novembre-décembre 1977, pp. 33-36.

174 Poupon (J.) "L'aménagement et l'amélioration des parcours forestiers au Maroc—1st partie" *Forêt Méditerranéenne*, tome I, no. 2, pp. 141-50.

175 Price (W. A.) "Nutrition and physical degeneration" Price-Pottenger Foundation, Santa Monica, Calif., 1945.

176 Provent (A.) & Ravignan (F. de) "Le nouvel ordre de la faim" Éd. du Seuil, Paris, 1977, p. 150.

177 Ramaut (Dr. J. L.) "Pesticides, biocénoses et chaînes trophiques" *Les Naturalistes Belges*, tome 46, no. 8, octobre 1965, pp. 348-91; no. 9, novembre 1965, pp. 421-38.

178 Ravignan (F. de) "Le nouvel ordre de la faim" Éd. du Seuil, Paris, 1971.

179 Ravignan (F. de) "Un village du Niger devant les experts occidentaux" *Le Monde Diplomatique*, novembre 1977, pp. 6-7.

180 Reddy (A. K. N.) "Critères pour la sélection des techniques" *Nouvelles de l'Écodéveloppement*, no. 7, décembre 1978, pp. 12-13.

181 Reddy (A. K. N.) "The Trojan Horse" *Cérès*, no. 50, March-April 1976, pp. 42-43.

182 Riding (A.) "Cotton Farmers in Guatemala Bombard Land with Pesticides" *International Herald Tribune*, 17 November 1977. Un résumé en francais de cet article se trouve dans *Nouvelles de l'Écodéveloppement*, no. 4, février 1978, p. 72.

183 Rogers (B.) "Mécanisation: pour hommes seulement" *Cérès*, no. 62, mars-avril 1978, pp. 12-14.

184 Roig (A.) "Dictionnaire des polluants alimentaires" Éd. de la Vie Claire (CEVIC), Mandres les Roses (France), 1973, p. 389.

185 Roig (A.) "Dictionnaire des polluants alimentaires— Supplément de mise à jour au 1 janvier 1977" Éd. CEVIC, 1977, p. 145.

186 Roy (P.) "Des maladies mystérieuses" *Mazingira, the International Journal of Environment and Development*, Tyrooly International Publishing Ltd., Dublin, Ireland, no. 6, 1978, pp. 74-77.

187 Sachs (I.) "Écodévelopper" *Cérès*, novembre-décembre 1974.

188 Sallenave (P.) "Cuisine et vitalité au Viet-Nam" *L'Alimentation Normale*, no. 21-22, AFRAN, Paris, 1959.

189 Samuel (A.) "Pourquoi la famine?" *Croissance des Jeunes Nations*, no. 215, mars 1980, pp. 19-26.

190 Sankale (M.); Satge (P.); Toury (J.); & Vuylsteke (S.) "Alimentation et pathologie nutritionnelle en Afrique Noire" Éd. Maloine, Paris, 1974.

191 Saouma (E.) "Introduction du thème: Promotion de l'usage rationnel des ressources naturelles" Symposium sur les relations mutuelles entre les ressources naturelles, l'environnement, la population et le développement, Stockholm, 6-11 août 1979, FAO, 1979, p. 12.

192 Scharpf (M. C.) & Aubert (C.) "Les engrais azotés ont une action défavorable sur la qualité nutritive des végétaux" février 1976, p. 15 in "Encyclopédie Permanente d'Agriculture Biologique," Éd. Debard, Paris, 1974-1976.

193 Schnell (R.) "Plantes alimentaires et vie agricole de l'Afrique Noire" Éd. Larose, Paris, 1957.

194 Shneour (E.) *The Malnourished Mind*, Doubleday, New York, 1974, pp. 98-100.

195 Shuphan (W.) *Nutritional Values in Crops and Plants*, Faber and Faber, London, 1965.

196 Smith (R. B. L.) "Une expérience de stockage du paddy en Thaïlande" *Appropriate Technology*, no. 9, p. 1.

197 Stanley (B.) "La préservation du grain" *Le CRDI explore*, vol. 5, no. 1, 1976.

198 Steinkraus (K. H.) *Handbook of Indigenous Fermented Foods*, Marcel Dekker, 1983.

199 Strahm (R. H.) "Pourquoi sont-ils si pauvres?" *A la Baconnière/La Déclaration de Berne*, Neuchâtel, 1977, p. 147.

200 Taylor (G. R.) *The Doomsday Book*, Thames and Hudson Ltd., London, 1970, pp. 89-91.

201 Taylor (T. A.) "Les associations culturales, moyen de lutte contre les parasites des plantes en Afrique Tropicale" *Environnement Africain*, vol. II, novembre 1977, pp. 113-20.

202 Thery (D.) "Héritage et créativité du savoir écologique populaire comme facteurs de développement sous-utilisés" *Nouvelles de l'Écodéveloppement*, no. 10, septembre 1979, pp. 8-31.

203 Thianar N'Doye (Dr.) interview "La nutrition procède de la philosophie" *Cérès*, no. 73, janvier-février 1980, pp. 17-23.

204 Toury (J.) *Les légumes et les fruits*. ORANA, Dakar, Document A 21, ronéotypé.

205 Toutain (G.) "Une approche globale: l'écosystème saharien—Mise en valeur des oasis à palmeraies dattières" Polycopié, INRA—GRET, 1979, p. 21.

206 Toutain (G.) & Collombon (J. M.) "Oasis de la vallée du Draa (Sud Maroc)" *Les Quatre Saisons du Jardinage*, no. 4, septembre-octobre 1980, pp. 75-83.

207 Tremolieres (J.) "Les mirages de l'aide" *Jeune Afrique*, Dossier Bis, "La crise alimentaire mondiale" janvier-février 1975, pp. 130-32.

208 Truhaut (R.) & Viel (G.) "Qualité des aliments: problème des résidus de pesticides" *Bulletin Technique d'Information* du Ministère de l'Agriculture, no. 287, février-mars 1974, pp. 65-73.

209 Tual (A.) "Les changements de l'alimentation traditionnelle dans la région de Téhéran" Communication des Traditions au Séminaire International du 1st Festival des Traditions Populaires à Ispahan, 14 octobre 1977, p. 26.

210 Van Veen (A. C.) & Steinkraus (K. H.) "Nutritive Value and Wholesomeness of Fermented Food" *Journal of Agricultural and Food Chemistry*, vol. 18, no. 4, août 1970, p. 576.

211 Van Veen (A. G.); Graham (D. C. W.); & Steinkraus (K. H.) "Fermented rice, a food from Ecuador" Separata de Archivos Latinoamericanos de Nutricion, vol. XVIII, no. 4, décembre 1968.

212 Vargas (F. de) "Lait en poudre et techniques de vente" *Le Monde Diplomatique*, juillet 1976, p. 6.

213 Veiga (J. da) "Radiographie de la Révolution Verte" *L'Économiste du Tiers-Monde*, septembre-octobre 1977, pp. 38-40.

214 Viel (J. M.) "L'agriculture biologique en France" Thèse de Doctorat de 3d cycle, Université de Paris I (IEDES), 1978.

215 Vietmeyer (N. D.) "Pitié pour les plantes des pauvres gens" *Cérès*, no. 62, mars-avril 1978, pp. 23-27.

216 Vissac (B.) "Nouvelles orientations de la politique de recherche de l'INRA" Polycopié, p. 6.

217 Voorhoeve (J. J. C.) "Le trésor dans la poubelle" *Cérès*, no. 50, mars-avril 1976, pp. 48-50.

218 Vulliez (H.) "Au coeur du Rwanda, des villageois s'organisent" *Croissance des Jeunes Nations*, no. 222, novembre 1980, pp. 31-35.

219 Weir (D.) & Shapiro (M.) "Pesticides sans frontières" CETIM, Genève, 1982.

220 Wenger (E.) "Environnement et Tiers-Monde africain" *Le Mois en Afrique*, no. 102, Paris, 1974, pp. 36-37.

221 Annual report, Cochabamba Agrobiology Project, F. Augstburger, 1981, Swiss Foundation for the Promotion of Biological Agriculture, Oberwill/BL, Simon I. Patino and Pro Bolivia Foundations, Geneva.

222 "Aspect écologique des problèmes phytosanitaires" *Purpan*, no. 99, avril-mai-juin 1976.

223 *Bulletin Technique d'Information* "La lutte biologique en agriculture" BTI, no. 332-333, septembre-octobre 1978, Paris.

224 "Les dangers du biberon" *Cérès*, mai-juin 1978.

225 "Dietary Goals for the United States" Selected Committee on Nutrition and Human Needs, U.S. Senate, Washington, D.C., 1977.

226 "L'emploi des engrais organiques en Inde" Ministère de l'Agriculture de New Delhi.

227 "Fertiliser naturellement" *Cérès*, mars-avril 1976.

228 "Le Handigodu syndrome" *Nouvelles de l'Écodéveloppement*, no. 4, février 1978.

229 "Mémento de l'adjoint technique des travaux ruraux" Ministère de la Coopération, Paris, 1977, pp. 316-18: Mesures à prendre à la suite d'aménagements hydrauliques.

230 "Monograph on Resistance of Agricultural Pests" FAO report, Washington, D.C., 1976, pp. 9-10.

231 National Academy of Sciences "Meeting Protein Needs of Infants and Preschool Children" National Research Council, Washington, D.C., 1961, pub. 843.

232 "Nutrition Canada" Enquête nationale, Ministère de la Santé, Ottawa, 1973.

233 "Les projets d'irrigation ignorent les problèmes de santé" *Cérès*, novembre-décembre 1979.

234 "Rapport sur l'État de Santé de la Population Française en 1972" INSERM, Paris, 1974.

235 "Report and Recommendations on Organic Farming" USDA, Washington, D.C., 1980.

236 "La seule solution est-elle l'engrais chimique?" *Environnement Africain*, vol. II, 4 & III, 1, novembre 1976.

INDEX

Page numbers in **boldface** indicate tables and charts.

Third World populations affected by pesticides, 62–63
types of diseases in irrigated areas, 89, 91–95
Herbicides, dioxin in, 68
Humus, 7, 23–24
I India
   Handigodu Syndrome in, 66–67
   kwashiorkor in, 141
   use of blue-green algae as a fertilizer in, 23–24
   village-scale biogas fertilizer plants in, 5, 6
   wells in, 98–99
Indians (American), levels of physical degeneration in, 131
Infant mortality and digestive infections, 125
Infections, 125, 151
Infectious diseases caused by protein deficiencies, 135
Insecticides
   amounts of, in milk, 55–56
   harmful effects of chemical, 10–12, 55–57
   plant-based, 3
   spread by air currents, 8, 9
   storage of crops and disadvantages of using, 43
   Third World populations and poisoning from, 62–63
   toxicity of, 58–60, **59**
   upsetting nature's balance with, 9
Insects
   microbiological methods for control of, 41–42
   resistance to pesticides, 2, 11–13
Intercropping, advantages of, 19–20
Irrigation
   effects on soil fertility, 89–90
   problems from dams, 95–98

   types of diseases in areas using, 89, 91–95
   use of wells in India, 98–99
   water-transmitted diseases, 93–95
Italy, dioxin poisoning in, 57, 68

K Kwashiorkor, 125, 135, 140, 141

L Lactic acid fermentation, 107, 109, 136–37, 146
Leaching, 6, 7, 19
Legumes
   vegetable protein in, 138–40
   vitamin B_{12} levels in sprouted, **149**
   vitamin C levels in sprouted, **150**
   yields of, 139
Leguminous plants
   associated cropping and, 20–22, **22**
   fermentation effects in, 113, **114**, 115–16
Life expectancy, eating habits and effects on, viii
Lindane, 43
Locust bean grains, fermentation of, 52–53

M Maize and associated cropping, 20–22, **22**
Malaria, 92, 132
Malathion, 12, 62–63
Malnutrition, 69–70, 125
Marasmus, 125
Mechanization of farms
   crop yields in United States and, 85–86, **86**
   disadvantages of, 83–84
   effects on the ecosystem, 84–85
   vs. small farms for developing countries, 81–82, 86–87
Mexico
   decline of breast feeding in, 125, **126**